THE OFFICIAL
PATIENT'S SOURCEBOOK
on

SCLERODERMA

JAMES N. PARKER, M.D.
AND PHILIP M. PARKER, PH.D., EDITORS

ICON Health Publications
ICON Group International, Inc.
4370 La Jolla Village Drive, 4th Floor
San Diego, CA 92122 USA

Printed in the United States of America.

Last digit indicates print number: 10 9 8 7 6 4 5 3 2 1

Publisher, Health Care: Tiffany LaRochelle
Editor(s): James Parker, M.D., Philip Parker, Ph.D.

Publisher's note: The ideas, procedures, and suggestions contained in this book are not intended as a substitute for consultation with your physician. All matters regarding your health require medical supervision. As new medical or scientific information becomes available from academic and clinical research, recommended treatments and drug therapies may undergo changes. The authors, editors, and publisher have attempted to make the information in this book up to date and accurate in accord with accepted standards at the time of publication. The authors, editors, and publisher are not responsible for errors or omissions or for consequences from application of the book, and make no warranty, expressed or implied, in regard to the contents of this book. Any practice described in this book should be applied by the reader in accordance with professional standards of care used in regard to the unique circumstances that may apply in each situation, in close consultation with a qualified physician. The reader is advised to always check product information (package inserts) for changes and new information regarding dose and contraindications before taking any drug or pharmacological product. Caution is especially urged when using new or infrequently ordered drugs, herbal remedies, vitamins and supplements, alternative therapies, complementary therapies and medicines, and integrative medical treatments.

Cataloging-in-Publication Data

Parker, James N., 1961-
Parker, Philip M, 1960-

The Official Patient's Sourcebook on Scleroderma: A Revised and Updated Directory for the Internet Age/James N. Parker and Philip M. Parker, editors
　　　　　p.　　　cm.
Includes bibliographical references, glossary and index.
ISBN: 0-597-82989-6
1. Scleroderma-Popular works.　　　I. Title.

Disclaimer

This publication is not intended to be used for the diagnosis or treatment of a health problem or as a substitute for consultation with licensed medical professionals. It is sold with the understanding that the publisher, editors, and authors are not engaging in the rendering of medical, psychological, financial, legal, or other professional services.

References to any entity, product, service, or source of information that may be contained in this publication should not be considered an endorsement, either direct or implied, by the publisher, editors or authors. ICON Group International, Inc., the editors, or the authors are not responsible for the content of any Web pages nor publications referenced in this publication.

Copyright Notice

If a physician wishes to copy limited passages from this sourcebook for patient use, this right is automatically granted without written permission from ICON Group International, Inc. (ICON Group). However, all of ICON Group publications are copyrighted. With exception to the above, copying our publications in whole or in part, for whatever reason, is a violation of copyright laws and can lead to penalties and fines. Should you want to copy tables, graphs or other materials, please contact us to request permission (e-mail: iconedit@san.rr.com). ICON Group often grants permission for very limited reproduction of our publications for internal use, press releases, and academic research. Such reproduction requires confirmed permission from ICON Group International Inc. **The disclaimer above must accompany all reproductions, in whole or in part, of this sourcebook.**

Dedication

To the healthcare professionals dedicating their time and efforts to the study of scleroderma.

Acknowledgements

The collective knowledge generated from academic and applied research summarized in various references has been critical in the creation of this sourcebook which is best viewed as a comprehensive compilation and collection of information prepared by various official agencies which directly or indirectly are dedicated to scleroderma. All of the *Official Patient's Sourcebooks* draw from various agencies and institutions associated with the United States Department of Health and Human Services, and in particular, the Office of the Secretary of Health and Human Services (OS), the Administration for Children and Families (ACF), the Administration on Aging (AOA), the Agency for Healthcare Research and Quality (AHRQ), the Agency for Toxic Substances and Disease Registry (ATSDR), the Centers for Disease Control and Prevention (CDC), the Food and Drug Administration (FDA), the Healthcare Financing Administration (HCFA), the Health Resources and Services Administration (HRSA), the Indian Health Service (IHS), the institutions of the National Institutes of Health (NIH), the Program Support Center (PSC), and the Substance Abuse and Mental Health Services Administration (SAMHSA). In addition to these sources, information gathered from the National Library of Medicine, the United States Patent Office, the European Union, and their related organizations has been invaluable in the creation of this sourcebook. Some of the work represented was financially supported by the Research and Development Committee at INSEAD. This support is gratefully acknowledged. Finally, special thanks are owed to Tiffany LaRochelle for her excellent editorial support.

About the Editors

James N. Parker, M.D.

Dr. James N. Parker received his Bachelor of Science degree in Psychobiology from the University of California, Riverside and his M.D. from the University of California, San Diego. In addition to authoring numerous research publications, he has lectured at various academic institutions. Dr. Parker is the medical editor for the *Official Patient's Sourcebook* series published by ICON Health Publications.

Philip M. Parker, Ph.D.

Philip M. Parker is the Eli Lilly Chair Professor of Innovation, Business and Society at INSEAD (Fontainebleau, France and Singapore). Dr. Parker has also been Professor at the University of California, San Diego and has taught courses at Harvard University, the Hong Kong University of Science and Technology, the Massachusetts Institute of Technology, Stanford University, and UCLA. Dr. Parker is the associate editor for the *Official Patient's Sourcebook* series published by ICON Health Publications.

About ICON Health Publications

In addition to scleroderma, *Official Patient's Sourcebooks* are available for the following related topics:

- The Official Patient's Sourcebook on Acne
- The Official Patient's Sourcebook on Acne Rosacea
- The Official Patient's Sourcebook on Atopic Dermatitis
- The Official Patient's Sourcebook on Behçet Syndrome
- The Official Patient's Sourcebook on Ehlers-danlos Syndrome
- The Official Patient's Sourcebook on Epidermolysis Bullosa
- The Official Patient's Sourcebook on Juvenile Rheumatoid Arthritis
- The Official Patient's Sourcebook on Lichen Sclerosus
- The Official Patient's Sourcebook on Lupus
- The Official Patient's Sourcebook on Lyme Disease
- The Official Patient's Sourcebook on Marfan Syndrome
- The Official Patient's Sourcebook on Osteogenesis Imperfecta
- The Official Patient's Sourcebook on Psoriasis
- The Official Patient's Sourcebook on Raynaud's Phenomenon
- The Official Patient's Sourcebook on Rheumatoid Arthritis
- The Official Patient's Sourcebook on Sjogren's Syndrome
- The Official Patient's Sourcebook on Vitiligo

To discover more about ICON Health Publications, simply check with your preferred online booksellers, including Barnes & Noble.com and Amazon.com which currently carry all of our titles. Or, feel free to contact us directly for bulk purchases or institutional discounts:

ICON Group International, Inc.
4370 La Jolla Village Drive, Fourth Floor
San Diego, CA 92122 USA
Fax: 858-546-4341
Web site: **www.icongrouponline.com/health**

Table of Contents

INTRODUCTION

Overview

Dr. C. Everett Koop, former U.S. Surgeon General, once said, "The best prescription is knowledge."[1] The Agency for Healthcare Research and Quality (AHRQ) of the National Institutes of Health (NIH) echoes this view and recommends that every patient incorporate education into the treatment process. According to the AHRQ:

> Finding out more about your condition is a good place to start. By contacting groups that support your condition, visiting your local library, and searching on the Internet, you can find good information to help guide your treatment decisions. Some information may be hard to find — especially if you don't know where to look.[2]

As the AHRQ mentions, finding the right information is not an obvious task. Though many physicians and public officials had thought that the emergence of the Internet would do much to assist patients in obtaining reliable information, in March 2001 the National Institutes of Health issued the following warning:

> The number of Web sites offering health-related resources grows every day. Many sites provide valuable information, while others may have information that is unreliable or misleading.[3]

---

[1] Quotation from http://www.drkoop.com.
[2] The Agency for Healthcare Research and Quality (AHRQ):
http://www.ahcpr.gov/consumer/diaginfo.htm.
[3] From the NIH, National Cancer Institute (NCI):
http://cancertrials.nci.nih.gov/beyond/evaluating.html.

Since the late 1990s, physicians have seen a general increase in patient Internet usage rates. Patients frequently enter their doctor's offices with printed Web pages of home remedies in the guise of latest medical research. This scenario is so common that doctors often spend more time dispelling misleading information than guiding patients through sound therapies. *The Official Patient's Sourcebook on Scleroderma* has been created for patients who have decided to make education and research an integral part of the treatment process. The pages that follow will tell you where and how to look for information covering virtually all topics related to scleroderma, from the essentials to the most advanced areas of research.

The title of this book includes the word "official." This reflects the fact that the sourcebook draws from public, academic, government, and peer-reviewed research. Selected readings from various agencies are reproduced to give you some of the latest official information available to date on scleroderma.

Given patients' increasing sophistication in using the Internet, abundant references to reliable Internet-based resources are provided throughout this sourcebook. Where possible, guidance is provided on how to obtain free-of-charge, primary research results as well as more detailed information via the Internet. E-book and electronic versions of this sourcebook are fully interactive with each of the Internet sites mentioned (clicking on a hyperlink automatically opens your browser to the site indicated). Hard copy users of this sourcebook can type cited Web addresses directly into their browsers to obtain access to the corresponding sites. Since we are working with ICON Health Publications, hard copy *Sourcebooks* are frequently updated and printed on demand to ensure that the information provided is current.

In addition to extensive references accessible via the Internet, every chapter presents a "Vocabulary Builder." Many health guides offer glossaries of technical or uncommon terms in an appendix. In editing this sourcebook, we have decided to place a smaller glossary within each chapter that covers terms used in that chapter. Given the technical nature of some chapters, you may need to revisit many sections. Building one's vocabulary of medical terms in such a gradual manner has been shown to improve the learning process.

We must emphasize that no sourcebook on scleroderma should affirm that a specific diagnostic procedure or treatment discussed in a research study, patent, or doctoral dissertation is "correct" or your best option. This sourcebook is no exception. Each patient is unique. Deciding on appropriate options is always up to the patient in consultation with their physician and healthcare providers.

Organization

This sourcebook is organized into three parts. Part I explores basic techniques to researching scleroderma (e.g. finding guidelines on diagnosis, treatments, and prognosis), followed by a number of topics, including information on how to get in touch with organizations, associations, or other patient networks dedicated to scleroderma. It also gives you sources of information that can help you find a doctor in your local area specializing in treating scleroderma. Collectively, the material presented in Part I is a complete primer on basic research topics for patients with scleroderma.

Part II moves on to advanced research dedicated to scleroderma. Part II is intended for those willing to invest many hours of hard work and study. It is here that we direct you to the latest scientific and applied research on scleroderma. When possible, contact names, links via the Internet, and summaries are provided. It is in Part II where the vocabulary process becomes important as authors publishing advanced research frequently use highly specialized language. In general, every attempt is made to recommend "free-to-use" options.

Part III provides appendices of useful background reading for all patients with scleroderma or related disorders. The appendices are dedicated to more pragmatic issues faced by many patients with scleroderma. Accessing materials via medical libraries may be the only option for some readers, so a guide is provided for finding local medical libraries which are open to the public. Part III, therefore, focuses on advice that goes beyond the biological and scientific issues facing patients with scleroderma.

Scope

While this sourcebook covers scleroderma, your doctor, research publications, and specialists may refer to your condition using a variety of terms. Therefore, you should understand that scleroderma is often considered a synonym or a condition closely related to the following:

- Familial Progressive Systemic Sclerosis
- Morphea
- Progressive Systemic Sclerosis

- Systemic Sclerosis

In addition to synonyms and related conditions, physicians may refer to scleroderma using certain coding systems. The International Classification of Diseases, 9th Revision, Clinical Modification (ICD-9-CM) is the most commonly used system of classification for the world's illnesses. Your physician may use this coding system as an administrative or tracking tool. The following classification is commonly used for scleroderma:[4]

- 710.1 systemic sclerosis

For the purposes of this sourcebook, we have attempted to be as inclusive as possible, looking for official information for all of the synonyms relevant to scleroderma. You may find it useful to refer to synonyms when accessing databases or interacting with healthcare professionals and medical librarians.

Moving Forward

Since the 1980s, the world has seen a proliferation of healthcare guides covering most illnesses. Some are written by patients or their family members. These generally take a layperson's approach to understanding and coping with an illness or disorder. They can be uplifting, encouraging, and highly supportive. Other guides are authored by physicians or other healthcare providers who have a more clinical outlook. Each of these two styles of guide has its purpose and can be quite useful.

As editors, we have chosen a third route. We have chosen to expose you to as many sources of official and peer-reviewed information as practical, for the purpose of educating you about basic and advanced knowledge as recognized by medical science today. You can think of this sourcebook as your personal Internet age reference librarian.

Why "Internet age"? All too often, patients diagnosed with scleroderma will log on to the Internet, type words into a search engine, and receive several Web site listings which are mostly irrelevant or redundant. These patients are left to wonder where the relevant information is, and how to obtain it. Since only the smallest fraction of information dealing with scleroderma is

---

[4] This list is based on the official version of the World Health Organization's 9th Revision, International Classification of Diseases (ICD-9). According to the National Technical Information Service, "ICD-9CM extensions, interpretations, modifications, addenda, or errata other than those approved by the U.S. Public Health Service and the Health Care Financing Administration are not to be considered official and should not be utilized. Continuous maintenance of the ICD-9-CM is the responsibility of the federal government."

even indexed in search engines, a non-systematic approach often leads to frustration and disappointment. With this sourcebook, we hope to direct you to the information you need that you would not likely find using popular Web directories. Beyond Web listings, in many cases we will reproduce brief summaries or abstracts of available reference materials. These abstracts often contain distilled information on topics of discussion.

While we focus on the more scientific aspects of scleroderma, there is, of course, the emotional side to consider. Later in the sourcebook, we provide a chapter dedicated to helping you find peer groups and associations that can provide additional support beyond research produced by medical science. We hope that the choices we have made give you the most options available in moving forward. In this way, we wish you the best in your efforts to incorporate this educational approach into your treatment plan.

The Editors

PART I: THE ESSENTIALS

ABOUT PART I

Part I has been edited to give you access to what we feel are "the essentials" on scleroderma. The essentials of a disease typically include the definition or description of the disease, a discussion of who it affects, the signs or symptoms associated with the disease, tests or diagnostic procedures that might be specific to the disease, and treatments for the disease. Your doctor or healthcare provider may have already explained the essentials of scleroderma to you or even given you a pamphlet or brochure describing scleroderma. Now you are searching for more in-depth information. As editors, we have decided, nevertheless, to include a discussion on where to find essential information that can complement what your doctor has already told you. In this section we recommend a process, not a particular Web site or reference book. The process ensures that, as you search the Web, you gain background information in such a way as to maximize your understanding.

CHAPTER 1. THE ESSENTIALS ON SCLERODERMA: GUIDELINES

Overview

Official agencies, as well as federally-funded institutions supported by national grants, frequently publish a variety of guidelines on scleroderma. These are typically called "Fact Sheets" or "Guidelines." They can take the form of a brochure, information kit, pamphlet, or flyer. Often they are only a few pages in length. The great advantage of guidelines over other sources is that they are often written with the patient in mind. Since new guidelines on scleroderma can appear at any moment and be published by a number of sources, the best approach to finding guidelines is to systematically scan the Internet-based services that post them.

The National Institutes of Health (NIH)[5]

The National Institutes of Health (NIH) is the first place to search for relatively current patient guidelines and fact sheets on scleroderma. Originally founded in 1887, the NIH is one of the world's foremost medical research centers and the federal focal point for medical research in the United States. At any given time, the NIH supports some 35,000 research grants at universities, medical schools, and other research and training institutions, both nationally and internationally. The rosters of those who have conducted research or who have received NIH support over the years include the world's most illustrious scientists and physicians. Among them are 97 scientists who have won the Nobel Prize for achievement in medicine.

---

[5] Adapted from the NIH: **http://www.nih.gov/about/NIHoverview.html**.

There is no guarantee that any one Institute will have a guideline on a specific disease, though the National Institutes of Health collectively publish over 600 guidelines for both common and rare diseases. The best way to access NIH guidelines is via the Internet. Although the NIH is organized into many different Institutes and Offices, the following is a list of key Web sites where you are most likely to find NIH clinical guidelines and publications dealing with scleroderma and associated conditions:

- Office of the Director (OD); guidelines consolidated across agencies available at **http://www.nih.gov/health/consumer/conkey.htm**

- National Library of Medicine (NLM); extensive encyclopedia (A.D.A.M., Inc.) with guidelines available at **http://www.nlm.nih.gov/medlineplus/healthtopics.html**

- National Institute of Arthritis and Musculoskeletal and Skin Diseases (NIAMS); fact sheets and guidelines at **http://www.nih.gov/niams/healthinfo/**

Among those listed above, the National Institute of Arthritis and Musculoskeletal and Skin Diseases (NIAMS) is especially noteworthy. The mission of NIAMS, a part of the National Institutes of Health (NIH), is to support research into the causes, treatment, and prevention of arthritis and musculoskeletal and skin diseases, the training of basic and clinical scientists to carry out this research, and the dissemination of information on research progress in these diseases. The National Institute of Arthritis and Musculoskeletal and Skin Diseases Information Clearinghouse is a public service sponsored by the NIAMS that provides health information and information sources. The NIAMS provides the following guideline concerning scleroderma.[6]

What Is Scleroderma?[7]

Derived from the Greek words "sklerosis," meaning hardness, and "derma," meaning skin, scleroderma literally means hard skin. Though it is often referred to as if it were a single disease, scleroderma is really a symptom of a group of diseases that involve the abnormal growth of connective tissue, which supports the skin and internal organs. It is sometimes used, therefore, as an umbrella term for these disorders. In some forms of scleroderma, hard,

---

[6]This and other passages are adapted from the NIH and NIAMS (**http://www.niams.nih.gov/hi/index.htm**). "Adapted" signifies that the text is reproduced with attribution, with some or no editorial adjustments.

[7] Adapted from the National Institute of Arthritis and Musculoskeletal and Skin Diseases (NIAMS): **http://www.niams.nih.gov/hi/topics/scleroderma/scleroderma.htm**.

tight skin is the extent of this abnormal process. In other forms, however, the problem goes much deeper, affecting blood vessels and internal organs, such as the heart, lungs, and kidneys.

Scleroderma is called both a rheumatic (roo-MA-tik) disease and a connective tissue disease. The term rheumatic disease refers to a group of conditions characterized by inflammation and/or pain in the muscles, joints, or fibrous tissue. A connective tissue disease is one that affects the major substances in the skin, tendons, and bones.

In this guideline we'll discuss the forms of scleroderma and the problems with each of them as well as diagnosis and disease management. We'll also take a look at what research is telling us about their possible causes and most effective treatments, and ways to help people with scleroderma live longer, healthier, and more productive lives.

What Are the Different Types of Scleroderma?

The group of diseases we call scleroderma falls into two main classes: localized scleroderma and systemic sclerosis. (Localized diseases affect only certain parts of the body; systemic diseases can affect the whole body.) Both groups include subgroups. Although there are different ways these groups and subgroups may be broken down or referred to (and your doctor may use different terms from what you see here), the following is a common way of classifying these diseases:

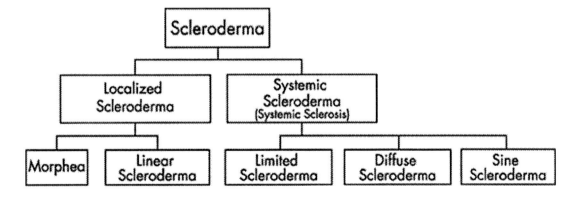

Localized Scleroderma

Localized types of scleroderma are those limited to the skin and related tissues and, in some cases, the muscle below. Internal organs are not affected by localized scleroderma, and localized scleroderma can never progress to the systemic form of the disease. Often, localized conditions improve or go away on their own over time, but the skin changes and damage that occur when the disease is active can be permanent. For some people, localized scleroderma is serious and disabling.

There are two generally recognized types of localized scleroderma:

- Morphea
- Linear scleroderma

Morphea

Morphea (mor-FEE-ah) comes from a Greek word that means "form" or "structure." The word refers to local patches of scleroderma. The first signs of the disease are reddish patches of skin that thicken into firm, oval-shaped areas. The center of each patch becomes ivory colored with violet borders. These patches sweat very little and have little hair growth. Patches appear most often on the chest, stomach, and back. Sometimes they appear on the face, arms, and legs.

Morphea can be either localized or generalized. Localized morphea limits itself to one or several patches, ranging in size from a half-inch to 12 inches in diameter. The condition sometimes appears on areas treated by radiation therapy. Some people have both morphea and linear scleroderma (described below). The disease is referred to as generalized morphea when the skin patches become very hard and dark and spread over larger areas of the body.

Regardless of the type, morphea generally fades out in 3 to 5 years; however, people are often left with darkened skin patches and, in rare cases, muscle weakness.

Linear Scleroderma

As suggested by its name, the disease has a single line or band of thickened and/or abnormally colored skin. Usually, the line runs down an arm or leg, but in some people it runs down the forehead. People sometimes use the French term *en coup de sabre*, or "sword stroke," to describe this highly visible line.

Systemic Scleroderma (Also Known As Systemic Sclerosis)

Systemic scleroderma, or systemic sclerosis, is the term for the disease that not only includes the skin, but also involves the tissues beneath to the blood vessels and major organs. Systemic sclerosis is typically broken down into diffuse and limited disease.

People with systemic sclerosis often have all or some of the symptoms that some doctors call CREST, which stands for the following:

- Calcinosis (KAL-sin-OH-sis): the formation of calcium deposits in the connective tissues, which can be detected by x ray. They are typically found on the fingers, hands, face, and trunk and on the skin above elbows and knees. When the deposits break through the skin, painful ulcers can result.

- Raynaud's (ray-NOHZ) phenomenon: a condition in which the small blood vessels of the hands and/or feet contract in response to cold or anxiety. As the vessels contract, the hands or feet turn white and cold, then blue. As blood flow returns, they become red. Fingertip tissues may suffer damage, leading to ulcers, scars, or gangrene.

- Esophageal (eh-SOFF-uh-GEE-ul) dysfunction: impaired function of the esophagus (the tube connecting the throat and the stomach) that occurs when smooth muscles in the esophagus lose normal movement. In the upper esophagus, the result can be swallowing difficulties; in the lower esophagus, the problem can cause chronic heartburn or inflammation.

- Sclerodactyly (SKLER-oh-DAK-till-ee): thick and tight skin on the fingers, resulting from deposits of excess collagen within skin layers. The condition makes it harder to bend or straighten the fingers. The skin may also appear shiny and darkened, with hair loss.

- Telangiectasias (tel-AN-jee-ek-TAY-zee-uhs): small red spots on the hands and face that are caused by the swelling of tiny blood vessels. While not painful, these red spots can create cosmetic problems.

Limited Scleroderma

Limited scleroderma typically comes on gradually and affects the skin only in certain areas: the fingers, hands, face, lower arms, and legs. Many people with limited disease have Raynaud's phenomenon for years before skin thickening starts. Others start out with skin problems over much of the body, which improves over time, leaving only the face and hands with tight, thickened skin. Telangiectasias and calcinosis often follow. Because of the predominance of CREST in people with limited disease, some doctors refer to limited disease as the CREST syndrome.

Diffuse Scleroderma

Diffuse scleroderma typically comes on suddenly. Skin thickening occurs quickly and over much of the body, affecting the hands, face, upper arms, upper legs, chest, and stomach in a symmetrical fashion (for example, if one arm or one side of the trunk is affected, the other is also affected). Some people may have more area of their skin affected than others. Internally, it can damage key organs such as the heart, lungs, and kidneys.

People with diffuse disease are often tired, lose appetite and weight, and have joint swelling and/or pain. Skin changes can cause the skin to swell, appear shiny, and feel tight and itchy.

The damage of diffuse scleroderma typically occurs over a few years. After the first 3 to 5 years, people with diffuse disease often enter a stable phase lasting for varying lengths of time. During this phase, skin thickness and appearance stay about the same. Damage to internal organs progresses little, if at all. Symptoms also subside: joint pain eases, fatigue lessens, and appetite returns.

Gradually, however, the skin starts to change again. Less collagen is made and the body seems to get rid of the excess collagen. This process, called "softening," tends to occur in reverse order of the thickening process: the last areas thickened are the first to begin softening. Some patients' skin returns to a somewhat normal state, while other patients are left with thin, fragile skin without hair or sweat glands. More serious damage to heart, lungs, or kidneys is unlikely to occur unless previous damage leads to more advanced deterioration.

People with diffuse scleroderma face the most serious long-term outlook if they develop severe kidney, lung, digestive, or heart problems. Fortunately, less than one-third of patients with diffuse disease develop these problems. Early diagnosis and continual and careful monitoring are important.

Sine Scleroderma

Some doctors break systemic sclerosis down into a third subset called systemic sclerosis sine (SEEN-ay, Latin for "without") scleroderma. Sine may resemble either limited or diffuse systemic sclerosis, causing changes in the lungs, kidneys, and blood vessels. However, there is one key difference between sine and other forms of systemic sclerosis: it does not affect the skin.

What Causes Scleroderma?

Although scientists don't know exactly what causes scleroderma, they are certain that people cannot catch it from or transmit it to others. Studies of twins suggest it is also not inherited. Scientists suspect that scleroderma comes from several factors that may include the following.

Abnormal Immune or Inflammatory Activity

Like many other rheumatic disorders, scleroderma is believed to be an autoimmune disease. An autoimmune disease is one in which the immune system, for unknown reasons, turns against one's own body.

In scleroderma, the immune system is thought to stimulate cells called fibroblasts to produce too much collagen. In scleroderma, collagen forms thick connective tissue that builds up around the cells of the skin and internal organs. In milder forms, the effects of this buildup are limited to the skin and blood vessels. In more serious forms, it also can interfere with normal functioning of skin, blood vessels, joints, and internal organs.

Genetic Makeup

While genes seem to put certain people at risk for scleroderma and play a role in its course, the disease is not passed from parent to child like some genetic diseases.

However, some research suggests that having children may increase a woman's risk of scleroderma. Scientists have learned that when a woman is pregnant, cells from her baby can pass through the placenta, enter her blood stream, and linger in her body--in some cases, for many years after the child's birth. Recently, scientists have found fetal cells from pregnancies of years past in the skin lesions of some women with scleroderma. They think that these cells, which are different from the woman's own cells, may either begin an immune reaction to the woman's own tissues or trigger a response by the woman's immune system to rid her body of those cells. Either way, the woman's healthy tissues may be damaged in the process. Further studies are needed to find out if fetal cells play a role in the disease.

Environmental Triggers

Research suggests that exposure to some environmental factors may trigger the disease in people who are genetically predisposed to it. Suspected triggers include viral infections, certain adhesive and coating materials, and organic solvents such as vinyl chloride or trichloroethylene. In the past, some people believed that silicone breast implants might have been a factor in developing connective tissue diseases such as scleroderma. But several studies have not shown evidence of a connection.

Hormones

By the middle to late childbearing years (ages 30 to 55), women develop scleroderma at a rate 7 to 12 times higher than men. Because of female predominance at this and all ages, scientists suspect that something distinctly feminine, such as the hormone estrogen, plays a role in the disease. So far, the role of estrogen or other female hormones has not been proven.

Who Gets Scleroderma?

Although scleroderma is more common in women, the disease also occurs in men and children. It affects people of all races and ethnic groups. However, there are some patterns by disease type. For example:

- Localized forms of scleroderma are more common in people of European descent than in African Americans.

- Morphea usually appears between the ages of 20 and 40.

- Linear scleroderma usually occurs in children or teenagers.

- Systemic scleroderma, whether limited or diffuse, typically occurs in people from 30 to 50 years old. It affects more women of African American than European descent.

Because scleroderma can be hard to diagnose and it overlaps with or resembles other diseases, scientists can only estimate how many cases there actually are. Estimates for the number of people in the United States with systemic sclerosis range from 40,000 to 165,000. By contrast, a survey that included all scleroderma-related disorders, including Raynaud's phenomenon, suggested a number between 250,000 and 992,500.

For some people, scleroderma (particularly the localized forms) is fairly mild and resolves with time. But for others, living with the disease and its effects day to day has a significant impact on their quality of life.

How Can Scleroderma Affect My Life?

Having a chronic disease can affect almost every aspect of your life, from family relationships to holding a job. For people with scleroderma, there may be other concerns about appearance or even the ability to dress, bathe, or handle the most basic daily tasks. Here are some areas in which scleroderma could intrude.

Appearance and Self-Esteem

Aside from the initial concerns about health and longevity, one of the first fears people with scleroderma have is how the disease will affect their appearance. Thick, hardened skin can be difficult to accept, particularly on the face. Systemic scleroderma may result in facial changes that eventually cause the opening to the mouth to become smaller and the upper lip to virtually disappear. Linear scleroderma may leave its mark on the forehead. Although these problems can't always be prevented, their effects may be minimized with proper treatment and skin care. Special cosmetics--and in some cases, plastic surgery--can help conceal scleroderma's damage.

Caring for Yourself

Tight, hard connective tissue in the hands can make it difficult to do what were once simple tasks, such as brushing your teeth and hair, pouring a cup of coffee, using a knife and fork, unlocking a door, or buttoning a jacket. If you have trouble using your hands, consult an occupational therapist, who can recommend new ways of doing things or devices to make tasks easier. Devices as simple as Velcro[8] fasteners and built-up brush handles can help you be more independent.

Family Relationships

Spouses, children, parents, and siblings may have trouble understanding why you don't have the energy to keep house, drive to soccer practice, prepare meals, and hold a job the way you used to. If your condition isn't that visible, they may even suggest you are just being lazy. On the other hand, they may be overly concerned and eager to help you, not allowing you to do the things you are able to do or giving up their own interests and activities to be with you. It's important to learn as much about your form of the disease as you can and share any information you have with your family. Involving them in counseling or a support group may also help them better understand the disease and how they can help you.

Sexual Relations

Sexual relationships can be affected when systemic scleroderma enters the picture. For men, the disease's effects on the blood vessels can lead to problems achieving an erection. In women, damage to the moisture-producing glands can cause vaginal dryness that makes intercourse painful. People of either sex may find they have difficulty moving the way they once did. They may be self-conscious about their appearance or afraid that their sexual partner will no longer find them attractive. With communication between partners, good medical care, and perhaps counseling, many of these changes can be overcome or at least worked around.

Pregnancy and Childbearing

In the past, women with systemic scleroderma were often advised not to have children. But thanks to better medical treatments and a better understanding of the disease itself, that advice is changing. (Pregnancy, for example, is not likely to be a problem for women with localized

---

[8] Brand names are provided as examples only, and their inclusion does not mean that these products are endorsed by the National Institutes of Health or any other Government agency. Also, if a particular brand name is not mentioned, this does not mean or imply that the product is unsatisfactory.

scleroderma.) Although blood vessel involvement in the placenta may cause babies of women with systemic scleroderma to be born early, many women with the disease can have safe pregnancies and healthy babies if they follow some precautions.

One of the most important pieces of advice is to wait a few years after the disease starts before attempting a pregnancy. During the first 3 years you are at the highest risk of developing severe problems of the heart, lungs, or kidneys that could be harmful to you and your unborn baby.

If you haven't developed organ problems within 3 years of the disease's onset, chances are you won't, and pregnancy should be safe. But it is important to have both your disease and your pregnancy monitored regularly. You'll probably need to stay in close touch with the doctor you typically see for your scleroderma as well as an obstetrician experienced in guiding high-risk pregnancies.

How Is Scleroderma Diagnosed?

Depending on your particular symptoms, a diagnosis of scleroderma may be made by a general internist, a dermatologist (a doctor who specializes in treating diseases of the skin, hair, and nails), an orthopaedist (a doctor who treats bone and joint disorders), a pulmonologist (lung specialist), or a rheumatologist (a doctor specializing in treatment of rheumatic diseases). A diagnosis of scleroderma is based largely on the medical history and findings from the physical exam. To make a diagnosis, your doctor will ask you a lot of questions about what has happened to you over time and about any symptoms you may be experiencing. Are you having a problem with heartburn or swallowing? Are you often tired or achy? Do your hands turn white in response to anxiety or cold temperatures?

Once your doctor has taken a thorough medical history, he or she will perform a physical exam. Finding one or more of the following factors can help the doctor diagnose a certain form of scleroderma:

- Changed skin appearance and texture, including swollen fingers and hands and tight skin around the hands, face, mouth, or elsewhere.

- Calcium deposits developing under the skin.

- Changes in the tiny blood vessels (capillaries) at the base of the fingernails.

- Thickened skin patches.

Finally, your doctor may order lab tests to help confirm a suspected diagnosis. At least two proteins, called antibodies, are commonly found in the blood of people with scleroderma:

- Antitopoisomerase-1 or Anti-Scl-70 antibodies appear in the blood of up to 40 percent of people with diffuse systemic sclerosis.

- Anticentromere antibodies are found in the blood of as many as 90 percent of people with limited systemic sclerosis.

A number of other scleroderma-specific antibodies can occur in people with scleroderma, although less frequently. When present, however, they are helpful in clinical diagnosis.

Because not all people with scleroderma have these antibodies and because not all people with the antibodies have scleroderma, lab test results alone cannot confirm the diagnosis.

In some cases, your doctor may order a skin biopsy (the surgical removal of a small sample of skin for microscopic examination) to aid in or help confirm a diagnosis. However, skin biopsies, too, have their limitations: biopsy results cannot distinguish between localized and systemic disease, for example.

Diagnosing scleroderma is easiest when a person has typical symptoms and rapid skin thickening. In other cases, a diagnosis may take months, or even years, as the disease unfolds and reveals itself and as the doctor is able to rule out some other potential causes of the symptoms. In some cases, a diagnosis is never made, because the symptoms that prompted the visit to the doctor go away on their own.

What Other Conditions Can Look Like Scleroderma?

Symptoms similar to those seen in scleroderma can occur with a number of other diseases. Some of the most common scleroderma look-alikes are listed below.

Eosinophilic Fasciitis (EF)

Eosinophilic fasciitis (EF) (EE-oh-SIN-oh-FIL-ik fa-shi-EYE-tis) is a disease that involves the fascia (FA-shuh), the thin connective tissue around the muscles, particularly those of the forearms, arms, legs, and trunk. EF causes the muscles to become encased in collagen, the fibrous protein that makes up tissue such as the skin and tendons. Permanent shortening of the muscles and tendons, called contractures, may develop, sometimes causing disfigurement and problems with joint motion and function. EF may begin after hard physical exertion. The disease usually fades away after several years, but people sometimes have relapses. Although the upper layers of the skin are not thickened in EF, the thickened fascia may cause the skin to look somewhat like the tight, hard skin of scleroderma. A skin biopsy easily distinguishes between the two.

Undifferentiated Connective Tissue Disease (UCTD)

Undifferentiated connective tissue disease (UCTD) is a diagnosis for patients who have some signs and symptoms of various related diseases, but not enough symptoms of any one disease to make a definite diagnosis. In other words, their condition hasn't "differentiated" into a particular connective tissue disease. In time, UCTD can go in one of three directions: it can change into a systemic disease such as systemic sclerosis, systemic lupus erythematosus, or rheumatoid arthritis; it can remain undifferentiated; or it can improve spontaneously.

Overlap Syndromes

Overlap syndromes a disease combination in which patients have symptoms and lab findings characteristic of two or more conditions.

At other times, symptoms resembling those of scleroderma can be the result of an unrelated disease or condition. For example:

- Skin thickening on the fingers and hands also appears with diabetes, mycosis fungoides, amyloidosis, and adult celiac disease. It can also result from hand trauma.

- Generalized skin thickening may occur with scleromyxedema, graft-versus-host disease, porphyria cutanea tarda, and human adjuvant disease.

- Internal organ damage, similar to that seen in systemic sclerosis, may instead be related to primary pulmonary hypertension, idiopathic pulmonary fibrosis, or collagenous colitis.

- Raynaud's phenomenon also appears with atherosclerosis or systemic lupus erythematosus or in the absence of underlying disease.

An explanation of most of these other diseases is beyond the scope of this guideline. What's important to understand, however, is that scleroderma isn't always easy to diagnose; it may take time for you and your doctor to establish a diagnosis. And while having a definite diagnosis may be helpful, knowing the precise form of your disease is not needed to receive proper treatment.

How Is Scleroderma Treated?

Because scleroderma can affect many different organs and organ systems, you may have several different doctors involved in your care. Typically, care will be managed by a rheumatologist, a specialist who treats people with diseases of the joints, bones, muscles, and immune system. Your rheumatologist may refer you to other specialists, depending on the specific problems you are having: for example, a dermatologist for the treatment of skin symptoms, a nephrologist for kidney complications, a cardiologist for heart complications, a gastroenterologist for problems of the digestive tract, and a pulmonary specialist for lung involvement.

In addition to doctors, professionals like nurse practitioners, physician assistants, physical or occupational therapists, psychologists, and social workers may play a role in your care. Dentists, orthodontists, and even speech therapists can treat oral complications that arise from thickening of tissues in and around the mouth and on the face.

Currently, there is no treatment that controls or stops the underlying problem--the overproduction of collagen--in all forms of scleroderma. Thus, treatment and management focus on relieving symptoms and limiting damage. Your treatment will depend on the particular problems you are having. Some treatments will be prescribed or given by your physician. Others are things you can do on your own.

Here are some of the potential problems that can occur in systemic scleroderma and the medical and nonmedical treatments for them. (These problems do not occur as a result or complication of localized scleroderma.)[9]

---

[9] Note: This is not a complete listing of problems or their treatments. Different people experience different problems with scleroderma and not all treatments work equally well for all people. Work with your doctor to find the best treatment for your specific symptoms.

Raynaud's Phenomenon

One of the most common problems associated with scleroderma, Raynaud's phenomenon can be uncomfortable and can lead to painful skin ulcers on the fingertips. Smoking makes the condition worse.

The following measures may make you more comfortable and help prevent problems:

- Don't smoke! Smoking narrows the blood vessels even more and makes Raynaud's phenomenon worse.

- Dress warmly, with special attention to hands and feet. Dress in layers and try to stay indoors during cold weather.

- Use biofeedback (to control various body processes that are not normally thought of as being under conscious control) and relaxation exercises.

- For severe cases, speak to your doctor about prescribing drugs called calcium channel blockers, such as nifedipine (Procardia), which can open up small blood vessels and improve circulation. Other drugs are in development and may become available in the future.

- If Raynaud's leads to skin sores or ulcers, increasing your dose of calcium channel blockers (under the direction of your doctor ONLY) may help. You can also protect skin ulcers from further injury or infection by applying nitroglycerine paste or antibiotic cream. Severe ulcerations on the fingertips can be treated with bioengineered skin.

More than 70 percent of people with scleroderma first notice this problem when their fingers turn cold or blue, typically in response to cold temperatures or emotional distress. Raynaud's phenomenon, as the condition is called, may precede scleroderma by years. In many people, however, Raynaud's phenomenon is unrelated to scleroderma, but may signal damage to the blood vessels supplying the hands arising from such conditions as occupational injuries (from using jackhammers, for example), trauma, excessive smoking, circulatory problems, and drug use or exposure to toxic substances. For some people, cold fingers (and toes) are the extent of the problem and are little more than a nuisance. For others, the condition can worsen and lead to puffy fingers, finger ulcers, and other complications that require aggressive treatment.

Stiff, Painful Joints

In diffuse systemic sclerosis, hand joints can stiffen because of hardened skin around the joints or inflammation of the joints themselves. Other joints can also become stiff and swollen. The following may help:

- Exercise regularly. Ask your doctor or physical therapist about an exercise plan that will help you increase and maintain range of motion in affected joints. Swimming can help maintain muscle strength, flexibility, and joint mobility.

- Use acetaminophen or an over-the-counter or prescription nonsteroidal anti-inflammatory drug, as recommended by your doctor, to help relieve joint or muscle pain. If pain is severe, speak to a rheumatologist about the possibility of prescription-strength drugs to ease pain and inflammation.

- Learn to do things in a new way. A physical or occupational therapist can help you learn to perform daily tasks, such as lifting and carrying objects or opening doors, in ways that will put less stress on tender joints.

Skin Problems

When too much collagen builds up in the skin, it crowds out sweat and oil glands, causing the skin to become dry and stiff. If your skin is affected, you may need to see a dermatologist. To ease dry skin, try the following:

- Apply oil-based creams and lotions frequently, and always right after bathing.

- Apply sunscreen before you venture outdoors, to protect against further damage by the sun's rays.

- Use humidifiers to moisten the air in your home in colder winter climates. (Clean humidifiers often to stop bacteria from growing in the water.)

- Avoid very hot baths and showers, as hot water dries the skin.

- Avoid harsh soaps, household cleaners, and caustic chemicals, if at all possible. If that's not possible, be sure to wear rubber gloves when you use such products.

- Exercise regularly. Exercise, especially swimming, stimulates blood circulation to affected areas.

Dry Mouth and Dental Problems

Dental problems are common in people with scleroderma for a number of reasons: tightening facial skin can make the mouth opening smaller and narrower, which makes it hard to care for teeth; dry mouth due to salivary gland damage speeds up tooth decay; and damage to connective tissues in the mouth can lead to loose teeth. You can avoid tooth and gum problems in several ways:

- Brush and floss your teeth regularly. (If hand pain and stiffness make this difficult, consult your doctor or an occupational therapist about specially made toothbrush handles and devices to make flossing easier.)

- Have regular dental checkups. Contact your dentist immediately if you experience mouth sores, mouth pain, or loose teeth.

- If decay is a problem, ask your dentist about fluoride rinses or prescription toothpastes that remineralize and harden tooth enamel.

- Consult a physical therapist about facial exercises to help keep your mouth and face more flexible.

- Keep your mouth moist by drinking plenty of water, sucking ice chips, using sugarless gum and hard candy, and avoiding mouthwashes with alcohol. If dry mouth still bothers you, ask your doctor about a saliva substitute or a prescription medication called pilocarpine hydrochloride (Salagen) that can stimulate the flow of saliva.

Gastrointestinal (GI) Problems

Systemic sclerosis can affect any part of the digestive system. As a result, you may experience problems such as heartburn, difficulty swallowing, early satiety (the feeling of being full after you've barely started eating), or intestinal complaints such as diarrhea, constipation, and gas. In cases where the intestines are damaged, your body may have difficulty absorbing nutrients from food. Although GI problems are diverse, here are some things that might help at least some of the problems you have:

- Eat small, frequent meals.

- Raise the head of your bed with blocks, and stand or sit for at least an hour (preferably two or three) after eating to keep stomach contents from backing up into the esophagus.

- Avoid late-night meals, spicy or fatty foods, and alcohol and caffeine, which can aggravate GI distress.

- Chew foods well and eat moist, soft foods. If you have difficulty swallowing or if your body doesn't absorb nutrients properly, your doctor may prescribe a special diet.

- Ask your doctor about prescription medications for problems such as diarrhea, constipation, and heartburn. Some drugs called proton pump inhibitors are highly effective against heartburn. Oral antibiotics may stop bacterial overgrowth in the bowel that can be a cause of diarrhea in some people with systemic sclerosis.

Lung damage

About 10 to 15 percent of people with systemic sclerosis develop severe lung disease, which comes in two forms: pulmonary fibrosis (hardening or scarring of lung tissue because of excess collagen) and pulmonary hypertension (high blood pressure in the artery that carries blood from the heart to the lungs). Treatment for the two conditions is different.

- Pulmonary fibrosis may be treated with drugs that suppress the immune system such as cyclophosphamide (Cytoxan) or azathioprine (Imuran), along with low doses of corticosteroids.

- Pulmonary hypertension may be treated with drugs that dilate the blood vessels such as prostacyclin (Iloprost).

Regardless of the problem or its treatment, your role in the treatment process is essentially the same. To minimize lung complications, work closely with your medical team. Do the following:

- Watch for signs of lung disease, including fatigue, shortness of breath or difficulty breathing, and swollen feet. Report these symptoms to your doctor.

- Have your lungs closely checked, using standard lung-function tests, during the early stages of skin thickening. These tests, which can find problems at the earliest and most treatable stages, are needed because lung damage can occur even before you notice any symptoms.

- Get regular flu and pneumonia vaccines as recommended by your doctor. Contracting either illness could be dangerous for a person with lung disease.

Heart Problems

About 15 to 20 percent of people with systemic sclerosis develop heart problems, including scarring and weakening of the heart (cardiomyopathy), inflamed heart muscle (myocarditis), and abnormal heart beat (arrhythmia). All of these problems can be treated. Treatment ranges from drugs to surgery, and varies depending on the nature of the condition.

Kidney Problems

About 15 to 20 percent of people with diffuse systemic sclerosis develop severe kidney problems, including loss of kidney function. Because uncontrolled high blood pressure can quickly lead to kidney failure, it's important that you take measures to minimize the problem. Things you can do:

- Check your blood pressure regularly and, if you find it to be high, call your doctor right away.

- If you have kidney problems, take your prescribed medications faithfully. In the past two decades, drugs known as ACE (angiotensin-converting enzyme) inhibitors, including captopril (Capoten), enalapril (Vasotec), and quinapril (Accupril), have made scleroderma-related kidney failure a less-threatening problem than it was in the past. But for these drugs to work, you must take them.

Cosmetic Problems

Even if scleroderma doesn't cause any lasting physical disability, its effects on the skin's appearance--particularly on the face--can take their toll on your self-esteem. Fortunately, there are procedures to correct some of the cosmetic problems scleroderma causes.

- The appearance of telangiectasias, small red spots on the hands and face caused by swelling of tiny blood vessels beneath the skin, may be lessened or even eliminated with the use of guided lasers.

- Facial changes of localized scleroderma, such as the en coup de sabre that may run down the forehead in people with linear scleroderma, may be corrected through cosmetic surgery. (However, such surgery is not appropriate for areas of the skin where the disease is active.)

How Can I Play a Role in My Health Care?

Although your doctors direct your treatment, you are the one who must take your medicine regularly, follow your doctor's advice, and report any problems promptly. In other words, the relationship between you and your doctors is a partnership, and you are the most important partner. Here's what you can do to make the most of this important role:

Get Educated

Knowledge is your best defense against this disease. Learn as much as you can about scleroderma, both for your own benefit and to educate the people in your support network.

Seek Support

Recruit family members, friends, and coworkers to build a support network. This network will help you get through difficult times, such as:

- When you are in pain;
- When you feel angry, sad, or afraid;
- When you're depressed.

Also, look for a scleroderma support group in your community by calling a national scleroderma organization. If you can't find a support group, you might want to consider organizing one.

Assemble a Healthcare Team

You and your doctors will lead the team. Other members may include physical and occupational therapists, a psychologist or social worker, a dentist, and a pharmacist.

Be Patient

Understand that a final diagnosis can be difficult and may take a long time. Find a doctor with experience treating people with systemic and localized scleroderma. Then, even if you don't yet have a diagnosis, you will get understanding and the right treatment for your symptoms.

Speak Up

When you have problems or notice changes in your condition, don't feel too self-conscious to speak up during your appointment or even call your doctor or another member of your health care team. No problem is too small to inquire about, and early treatment for any problem can make the disease more manageable for you and your health care team.

Don't Accept Depression

While it's understandable that a person with a chronic illness like scleroderma would become depressed, don't accept depression as a normal consequence of your condition. If depression makes it hard for you to function well, don't hesitate to ask your health care team for help. You may benefit from speaking with a psychologist or social worker or from using one of the effective medications on the market.

Learn Coping Skills

Skills like meditation, calming exercises, and relaxation techniques may help you cope with emotional difficulties as well as help relieve pain and fatigue. Ask a member of your health care team to teach you these skills or to refer you to someone who can.

Ask the Experts

If you have problems doing daily activities, from brushing your hair and teeth to driving your car, consult an occupational or physical therapist. They have more helpful hints and devices than you can probably imagine. Social workers can often help resolve financial and insurance matters.

Is Research Close to Finding a Cure?

No one can say for sure when--or if--a cure will be found. But research is providing the next best thing -- better ways to treat symptoms, prevent organ damage, and improve the quality of life for people with scleroderma. In the past two decades, multidisciplinary research has also provided new clues to understanding the disease, which is an important step toward prevention or cure.

Leading the way in funding for this research is the National Institute of Arthritis and Musculoskeletal and Skin Diseases (NIAMS), a part of the National Institutes of Health (NIH). Other sources of funding for scleroderma research include pharmaceutical companies and organizations such as the Scleroderma Foundation, the Scleroderma Research Foundation, and the Arthritis Foundation. Scientists at universities and medical centers throughout the United States conduct much of this research.

Studies of the immune system, genetics, cell biology, and molecular biology have helped reveal the causes of scleroderma, improve existing treatment, and create entirely new treatment approaches.

Research advances in recent years that have led to a better understanding of and/or treatment for the diseases include:

- The use of a hormone produced in pregnancy to soften skin lesions. Early studies suggest relaxin, a hormone that helps a woman's body to stretch to meet the demands of a growing pregnancy and delivery, may soften the connective tissues of women with scleroderma. The hormone is believed to work by blocking fibrosis, or the development of fibrous tissue between the body's cells.

- Finding a gene associated with scleroderma in Oklahoma Choctaw Native Americans. Scientists believe the gene, which codes for a protein called fibrillin-1, may put people at risk for the disease.

- The use of the drug Iloprost for pulmonary hypertension. This drug has increased the quality of life and life expectancy for people with this dangerous form of lung damage.

- The use of the drug cyclophosphamide (Cytoxan) for lung fibrosis. One recent study suggested that treating lung problems early with this immunosuppressive drug may help prevent further damage and increase chances of survival.

- The increased use of ACE inhibitors for scleroderma-related kidney problems. For the past two decades, ACE inhibitors have greatly reduced the risk of kidney failure in people with scleroderma. Now there is evidence that use of ACE inhibitors can actually heal the kidneys of people on dialysis for scleroderma-related kidney failure. As many as half of people who continue ACE inhibitors while on dialysis may be able to go off dialysis in 12 to 18 months.

Other studies are examining the following:

- Changes in the tiny blood vessels of people with scleroderma. By studying these changes, scientists hope to find the cause of cold sensitivity in Raynaud's phenomenon and how to control the problem.

- Immune system changes (and particularly how those changes affect the lungs) in people with early diffuse systemic sclerosis.

- The role of blood vessel malfunction, cell death, and autoimmunity in scleroderma.

- Skin changes in laboratory mice in which a genetic defect prevents the breakdown of collagen, leading to thick skin and patchy hair loss. Scientists hope that by studying these mice, they can answer many questions about skin changes in scleroderma.

- The effectiveness of various treatments, including (1) methotrexate, a drug commonly used for rheumatoid arthritis and some other inflammatory forms of arthritis; (2) collagen peptides administered orally; (3) halofugione, a drug that inhibits the synthesis of type I collagen, which is the primary component of connective tissue; (4) ultraviolet light therapy for localized forms of scleroderma; and (5) stem cell transfusions, a form of bone marrow transplant that uses a patient's own cells, for early diffuse systemic sclerosis.

Scleroderma research continues to advance as scientists and doctors learn more about how the disease develops and its underlying mechanisms.

Recently, the NIAMS funded a Specialized Center of Research (SCOR) in scleroderma at the University of Texas-Houston. SCOR scientists are conducting laboratory and clinical research on the disease. The SCOR approach allows researchers to translate basic science findings quickly into improved treatment and patient care.

More Questions? Count on More Answers

Scleroderma poses a series of challenges for both patients and their health care teams. The good news is that scientists, doctors, and other health care professionals continue to find new answers--ways to make earlier diagnoses and manage disease better. In addition, active patient support groups share with, care for, and educate each other. The impact of all of this activity is that people with scleroderma do much better and remain active far longer than they did 20 or 30 years ago. As for tomorrow, patients and the medical community will continue to push for longer, healthier, and more active lives for people with the diseases collectively known as scleroderma.

National Resources for Scleroderma

For more information, contact:

National Institute of Arthritis and Musculoskeletal and Skin Diseases Information Clearinghouse
NIAMS/National Institutes of Health
1 AMS Circle
Bethesda, MD 20892-3675
(301) 495-4484 or (877) 22-NIAMS (226-4267) (free of charge)
TTY: (301) 565-2966
Fax: (301) 718-6366
www.niams.nih.gov
This clearinghouse, a public service sponsored by the National Institute of Arthritis and Musculoskeletal and Skin Diseases (NIAMS), provides information about various forms of arthritis and rheumatic diseases. The clearinghouse distributes patient and professional education materials and also refers people to other sources of information.

American Academy of Dermatology
930 N. Meacham Road
P.O. Box 4014
Schaumburg, IL 60168-4014
(847) 330-0230
www.aad.org
This national professional association for dermatologists publishes a pamphlet on skin conditions and can also provide physician referrals.

American College of Rheumatology
1800 Century Place, Suite 250
Atlanta, GA 30345
(404) 633-3777
Fax: (404) 633-1870
www.rheumatology.org
This association provides referrals to doctors and health professionals who work on arthritis, rheumatic diseases, and related conditions. The association also provides educational materials and guidelines.

Scleroderma Foundation

12 Kent Way, #101

Byfield, MA 01922

(800) 722-HOPE (free of charge) or (978) 463-5843

Fax: (978) 463-5809

E-mail: sfinfo@scleroderma.org

www.scleroderma.org

The foundation publishes information on scleroderma and offers patient education seminars, support groups, physician referrals, and information hotlines.

Scleroderma Research Foundation

2320 Bath Street, Suite 315

Santa Barbara, CA 93105

(800) 441-CURE (2873) (free of charge) or (805) 563-9133

www.srfcure.org

The foundation's goal is to find a cure for scleroderma by funding and facilitating the most promising, highest quality research and by placing the disease and its need for a cure in the public eye. The foundation distributes patient handbooks and a twice yearly, research-related newsletter.

Arthritis Foundation

1330 West Peachtree Street

Atlanta, GA 30309

Call your local chapter (listed in the telephone directory), or (404) 872-7100 or (800) 283-7800 (free of charge)

www.arthritis.org

The foundation is a major voluntary organization devoted to supporting research on arthritis and other rheumatic diseases, such as scleroderma. It also provides up-to-date information on treatments, nutrition, alternative therapies, and self-management strategies. Chapters nationwide offer exercise programs, classes, support groups, physician referral services, and free literature.

More Guideline Sources

The guideline above on scleroderma is only one example of the kind of material that you can find online and free of charge. The remainder of this chapter will direct you to other sources which either publish or can help you find additional guidelines on topics related to scleroderma. Many of the guidelines listed below address topics that may be of particular relevance to your specific situation or of special interest to only some patients with scleroderma. Due to space limitations these sources are listed in a concise manner. Do not hesitate to consult the following sources by either using the Internet hyperlink provided, or, in cases where the contact information is provided, contacting the publisher or author directly.

Topic Pages: MEDLINEplus

For patients wishing to go beyond guidelines published by specific Institutes of the NIH, the National Library of Medicine has created a vast and patient-oriented healthcare information portal called MEDLINEplus. Within this Internet-based system are "health topic pages." You can think of a health topic page as a guide to patient guides. To access this system, log on to **http://www.nlm.nih.gov/medlineplus/healthtopics.html**. From there you can either search using the alphabetical index or browse by broad topic areas.

If you do not find topics of interest when browsing health topic pages, then you can choose to use the advanced search utility of MEDLINEplus at **http://www.nlm.nih.gov/medlineplus/advancedsearch.html**. This utility is similar to the NIH Search Utility, with the exception that it only includes material linked within the MEDLINEplus system (mostly patient-oriented information). It also has the disadvantage of generating unstructured results. We recommend, therefore, that you use this method only if you have a very targeted search.

The Combined Health Information Database (CHID)

CHID Online is a reference tool that maintains a database directory of thousands of journal articles and patient education guidelines on scleroderma and related conditions. One of the advantages of CHID over other sources is that it offers summaries that describe the guidelines available, including contact information and pricing. CHID's general Web site is **http://chid.nih.gov/**. To search this database, go to **http://chid.nih.gov/detail/detail.html**. In particular, you can use the advanced search options to look up pamphlets, reports, brochures, and information kits. The following was recently posted in this archive:

- **Scleroderma: An Overview**

    Source: Danvers, MA: Scleroderma Foundation. 2000. 6 p.

Contact: Available from Scleroderma Foundation. 12 Kent Way, Suite 101, Byfield, MA 01922. (800) 722-4673 or (978) 463-5843. Fax (978) 463-5809. E-mail: sfinfo@scleroderma.org. Website: www.scleroderma.org. Price: Single copy $1.00.

Summary: This pamphlet for people with scleroderma provides an overview of this autoimmune connective tissue disease that affects the skin and internal organs. It presents the features of the systemic and localized forms of scleroderma. In systemic scleroderma, the immune system causes damage to the small blood vessels and the collagen-producing cells located in the skin and throughout the body. Systemic scleroderma is categorized as limited or diffuse, although both forms are associated with internal organ damage. The limited form tends to have less severe organ problems than the diffuse form. The limited form is frequently referred to as the CREST form, which is an acronym that stands for calcinosis, Raynaud's phenomenon, esophageal dysfunction, sclerodactyly, and telangiectasias. Localized scleroderma affects the collagen producing cells in some of the areas of the skin and usually spares the internal organs and blood vessels. The pamphlet also answers questions about who gets scleroderma, whether genetic factors are involved, and how it is treated. It concludes with information on the mission of the Scleroderma Foundation.

- **What Causes Scleroderma?**

Source: Danvers, MA: Scleroderma Foundation. 2000. 6 p.

Contact: Available from Scleroderma Foundation. 12 Kent Way, Suite 101, Byfield, MA 01922. (800) 722-4673 or (978) 463-5843. Fax (978) 463-5809. E-mail: sfinfo@scleroderma.org. Website: www.scleroderma.org. Price: Single copy $1.00.

Summary: This pamphlet for people with scleroderma provides information on clinical and laboratory features of scleroderma that offer clues to the cause of this disease. Almost every patient with scleroderma has a condition known as Raynaud's phenomenon, which is associated with tissue damage and ulceration caused by low blood flow. Most people with scleroderma show evidence of an autoimmune reaction because immune cells, known as T-cells, are found in abnormal numbers in the tissues of patients with scleroderma. Almost all patients with scleroderma develop a fibrotic reaction in the tissues targeted in scleroderma. In addition, a genetic basis for scleroderma has been suggested by the fact that scleroderma occurs among patients whose family members are more likely to have other autoimmune diseases. The brochure uses these features of scleroderma to suggest a possible mechanism by which it occurs. In addition, it presents the mission of the Scleroderma Foundation.

- **Gastrointestinal Tract in Scleroderma**

  Source: Danvers, MA: Scleroderma Foundation. 1999. 6 p.

  Contact: Available from Scleroderma Foundation. 12 Kent Way, Suite 101, Byfield, MA 01922. (800) 722-4673 or (978) 463-5843. Fax (978) 463-5809. E-mail: sfinfo@scleroderma.org. Website: www.scleroderma.org. Price: Single copy $1.00.

  Summary: This pamphlet provides people who have scleroderma with information on its gastrointestinal tract manifestations. The pamphlet focuses on manifestations involving the mouth, esophagus, stomach, and small intestine and large intestines. People who have scleroderma may experience dry mouth, which may lead to impairment of early digestion and occurrence of dental caries and periodontitis. Involvement of the esophagus may cause heartburn, difficulty with swallowing, and aspiration. Stomach involvement occurs in only 10 percent of patients, but it can be associated with bloating, satiety, abdominal pain, nausea, and vomiting. Involvement of the small intestine may cause nausea, vomiting, bloating, diarrhea, and malabsorption, while muscle impairment of the large intestine may result in constipation, bloating, and diarrhea. The pamphlet also includes a glossary of terms. 1 figure.

- **Dental Care in Scleroderma**

  Source: Danvers, MA: Scleroderma Foundation. 1999. 6 p.

  Contact: Available from Scleroderma Foundation. 12 Kent Way, Suite 101, Byfield, MA 01922. (800) 722-4673 or (978) 463-5843. Fax (978) 463-5809. E-mail: sfinfo@scleroderma.org. Website: www.scleroderma.org. Price: Single copy $1.00.

  Summary: This pamphlet provides people who have scleroderma with information on dental care. Xerostomia, or dry mouth, and microstomia, or limited mouth opening, are two common problems associated with scleroderma. People who experience xerostomia are more susceptible to periodontal disease, dental caries, and yeast and bacterial infections. The pamphlet presents possible strategies for minimizing the problems associated with xerostomia, lists foods and substances to avoid, offers suggestions on eating, and discusses possible denture problems and solutions. Microstomia may lead to impairment of chewing and compromise the ability to perform routine oral hygiene. The pamphlet identifies special hygiene devices and techniques for microstomia.

- **Raynaud's Phenomenon**

  Source: Danvers, MA: Scleroderma Foundation. 1998. 6 p.

  Contact: Available from Scleroderma Foundation. 12 Kent Way, Suite 101, Byfield, MA 01922. (800) 722-4673 or (978) 463-5843. Fax (978) 463-5809. E-mail: sfinfo@scleroderma.org. Website: www.scleroderma.org. Price: Single copy $1.00.

  Summary: This pamphlet uses a question and answer format to provide people who have scleroderma with information on Raynaud's phenomenon. This condition, which consists of episodic attacks of paleness or blueness in the fingertips or toes, occurs in over 90 percent of people with scleroderma and is universal in the CREST form. This acronym stands for calcinosis, Raynaud's phenomenon, esophagitis, sclerodactyly, and telangiectasias. Raynaud's is strongly associated with the other features of this acronym. The pamphlet explains who develops Raynaud's, how a doctor evaluates a patient who has it and how it is treated. There is no specific blood test that identifies Raynaud's phenomenon, but common laboratory findings in people with the condition include an antinuclear antibody; rheumatoid factor; or antibodies to centromere, ribonucleoprotein, or DNA. The management of Raynaud's involves both drug and nondrug therapies. The pamphlet concludes with information on the mission of the Scleroderma Foundation.

- **Coping With Scleroderma**

  Source: Danvers, MA: Scleroderma Foundation. 1998. 8 p.

  Contact: Available from Scleroderma Foundation. 12 Kent Way, Suite 101, Byfield, MA 01922. (800) 722-4673 or (978) 463-5843. Fax (978) 463-5809. E-mail: sfinfo@scleroderma.org. Website: www.scleroderma.org. Price: Single copy $1.00.

  Summary: This pamphlet intended for people with scleroderma, focuses on adjusting to the disease. It discusses the emotional stages that people often go through before they acknowledge their changed lives. The initial stages involve waiting for and receiving the diagnosis. Subsequent stages may involve denying the reality of the disease, getting angry and depressed, bargaining, and finally accepting it. The pamphlet provides practical tips for coping with each stage and highlights some of the characteristics of people who have learned to cope with the disease. It concludes with information on the mission of the Scleroderma Foundation.

- **Scleroderma**

  Source: Atlanta, GA: Arthritis Foundation. 1997. 10 p.

  Contact: Available from Arthritis Foundation. P.O. Box 1616, Alpharetta, GA 30009-1616. (800) 207-8633. Fax (credit card orders only) (770) 442-9742. http://www.arthritis.org. Price: Single copy free from local Arthritis Foundation chapter (call 800-283-7800 for closest local chapter); bulk orders may be purchased from address above.

  Summary: This brochure for people with scleroderma uses a question and answer format to provide information on this rare, chronic disease, which affects women much more often than men. Although the cause is unknown, scientists know that a person with scleroderma produces too much collagen, which causes thickening and hardening of the skin and affects the functioning of internal organs. The brochure outlines the ways in which the various forms of scleroderma affect the body and it explains how the disease is diagnosed and treated. Treatment may consist of medication, exercise, joint and skin protection, and stress management. The brochure also provides information on the Arthritis Foundation.

- **Scleroderma Handbook**

  Source: Santa Barbara, CA: Scleroderma Research Foundation. 199x. 20 p.

  Contact: Available from Scleroderma Research Foundation. Pueblo Medical Commons, 2320 Bath Street, Suite 307, Santa Barbara, CA 93105. (800) 441-CURE or (805) 563-9133. Website: www.srfcure.org. Price: Single copy free.

  Summary: This booklet provides people who have scleroderma, a chronic, degenerative disease that causes overproduction of collagen in the body's connective tissue, with information on its symptoms, diagnosis, treatment, and prognosis. The booklet describes the cutaneous, vascular, and other manifestations of scleroderma; lists the common manifestations represented by the CREST acronym, and outlines general symptoms. The features of several types of scleroderma are described, especially systemic scleroderma and limited forms of scleroderma. Although no one specific test can accurately and definitively determine whether a patient has scleroderma, the nailfold capillary test is a useful clinical tool. Physicians commonly consulted for diagnosis and treatment include a rheumatologist, a dermatologist, and an internist. Other topics discussed are the importance of becoming one's own health advocate and obstacles to and progress in scleroderma research.

- **Localized Scleroderma**

  Source: Danvers, MA: Scleroderma Foundation. 1999. 8 p.

  Contact: Available from Scleroderma Foundation. 12 Kent Way, Suite 101, Byfield, MA 01922. (800) 722-4673 or (978) 463-5843. Fax (978) 463-5809. E-mail: sfinfo@scleroderma.org. Website: www.scleroderma.org. Price: Single copy $1.00.

  Summary: This pamphlet uses a question and answer format to provide people who have scleroderma with information on the nature and complications of localized scleroderma, as well as its treatment and prognosis. This condition, which has no known cause, is characterized by thickening of the skin from excessive collagen deposition. Localized scleroderma is limited to the skin and underlying muscle and tissue. Diagnosis is based on visual recognition and a skin biopsy, although several blood tests may be used to help determine how active the disease is and how extensive or prolonged it may become. There are four main types of localized scleroderma: morphea, generalized morphea, linear scleroderma, and en coup de sabre. The pamphlet describes their features and discusses the prognosis for patients who have each type. Several drugs may be used to help halt the spread of the disease, and various other treatments may be used to help the condition.

- **Handout on Health: Scleroderma**

  Source: Bethesda, MD: National Institute of Arthritis and Musculoskeletal and Skin Diseases (NIAMS) Information Clearinghouse. 2001. 48 p.

  Contact: Available from National Institute of Arthritis and Musculoskeletal and Skin Diseases (NIAMS) Information Clearinghouse. 1 AMS Circle, Bethesda, MD 20892-3675. (877) 226-4267 toll-free or (301) 495-4484. Fax (301) 718-6366. TTY (301) 565-2966. E-mail: NIAMSInfo@mail.nih.gov. Website: www.niams.nih.gov. Price: 1 to 25 free. Order Number: AR-113 HH (booklet), or AR-113L HH (large print fact sheet).

  Summary: This booklet uses a question and answer format to provide people who have scleroderma and their family members and friends with information on the types, symptoms, causes, diagnosis, and treatment of this disease. Scleroderma is a symptom of a group of diseases that involve the abnormal growth of connective tissue. It is classified as both a rheumatic disease and a connective tissue disease. The main types are localized scleroderma and systemic sclerosis. Localized scleroderma includes morphea and linear scleroderma. Systemic scleroderma, which is also known as systemic sclerosis, can be broken down into limited or diffuse scleroderma. Although the exact cause is unknown, scientists suspect that scleroderma is caused by several factors, including abnormal immune or inflammatory activity, genetic makeup, environmental triggers, and hormones. Scleroderma affects people of all races and ethnic groups, and it is more common in women. The disease can affect various aspects of life, including appearance and self esteem, self care, family relationships, sexual relations, and pregnancy and childbearing. Diagnosis is based on medical history, physical examination, and laboratory tests. Many conditions can mimic the symptoms of scleroderma, including eosinophilic fasciitis, undifferentiated connective tissue disease, and overlap syndromes. Management may involve many doctors. There is no treatment that controls or stops the underlying problem, so treatment and management focus on relieving symptoms and limiting damage. The booklet discusses the medical and nonmedical treatments for various problems that can occur in systemic scleroderma, including Raynaud's phenomenon; stiff and painful joints; skin problems; dry mouth and dental problems; gastrointestinal, heart, and kidney problems; lung damage; and cosmetic problems. Other topics includes ways people can manage their own health and current research aimed at understanding and treating scleroderma, particularly research supported by the National Institute of Arthritis and Musculoskeletal and Skin Diseases and other components of the National Institutes of Health. The booklet includes a glossary and list of national resources.

- **Scleroderma Fact Sheet**

  Source: Danvers, MA: Scleroderma Foundation. 199X. 2 p.

  Contact: Available from Scleroderma Foundation. 12 Kent Way, Suite 101, Byfield, MA 01922. (800) 722-4673 or (978) 463-5843. Fax (978) 463-5809. E-mail: sfinfo@scleroderma.org. Website: www.scleroderma.org. Price: $0.25.

  Summary: This fact sheet for people with scleroderma presents facts about this chronic, autoimmune connective tissue disease, which is also known as systemic sclerosis. It explains that scleroderma is a highly individualized disease with wide-ranging symptoms that may affect the skin or internal organs, but that as a general rule, scleroderma is not contagious, cancerous, or inherited. It answers questions on the number of people with scleroderma, what causes it, and how it is diagnosed. In addition, the fact sheet provides information on localized scleroderma and systemic sclerosis.

The National Guideline Clearinghouse™

The National Guideline Clearinghouse™ offers hundreds of evidence-based clinical practice guidelines published in the United States and other countries. You can search their site located at **http://www.guideline.gov** by using the keyword "scleroderma" or synonyms.

Healthfinder™

Healthfinder™ is an additional source sponsored by the U.S. Department of Health and Human Services which offers links to hundreds of other sites that contain healthcare information. This Web site is located at **http://www.healthfinder.gov**. Again, keyword searches can be used to find guidelines. The following was recently found in this database:

- **Handout on Health: Scleroderma**

    Summary: This booklet is for people who have scleroderma, as well as for their family members, friends, and others who want to find out more about the disease.

    Source: National Institute of Arthritis and Musculoskeletal and Skin Diseases, National Institutes of Health

    http://www.healthfinder.gov/scripts/recordpass.asp?RecordType=0&RecordID=6695

- **Scleroderma Fact Sheet**

    Summary: This consumer information mini-fact sheet provides basic information about this auto-immune disease of the connective tissue, generally classified as one of the rheumatic diseases.

    Source: Scleroderma Foundation

    http://www.healthfinder.gov/scripts/recordpass.asp?RecordType=0&RecordID=2433

- **Scleroderma Physician Referral List**

    Summary: Search by city, state, name, and specialty for a physician familiar with scleroderma.

    Source: Scleroderma Research Foundation

    http://www.healthfinder.gov/scripts/recordpass.asp?RecordType=0&RecordID=6825

- **Scleroderma Support Groups**

  Summary: Select a state to find a scleroderma support group in your area. A toll-free phone number is listed for further information if there is no support group in your area.

  Source: Scleroderma Foundation

  http://www.healthfinder.gov/scripts/recordpass.asp?RecordType=0&RecordID=2659

The NIH Search Utility

After browsing the references listed at the beginning of this chapter, you may want to explore the NIH Search Utility. This allows you to search for documents on over 100 selected Web sites that comprise the NIH-WEB-SPACE. Each of these servers is "crawled" and indexed on an ongoing basis. Your search will produce a list of various documents, all of which will relate in some way to scleroderma. The drawbacks of this approach are that the information is not organized by theme and that the references are often a mix of information for professionals and patients. Nevertheless, a large number of the listed Web sites provide useful background information. We can only recommend this route, therefore, for relatively rare or specific disorders, or when using highly targeted searches. To use the NIH search utility, visit the following Web page: **http://search.nih.gov/index.html**.

NORD (The National Organization of Rare Disorders, Inc.)

NORD provides an invaluable service to the public by publishing, for a nominal fee, short yet comprehensive guidelines on over 1,000 diseases. NORD primarily focuses on rare diseases that might not be covered by the previously listed sources. NORD's Web address is **www.rarediseases.org**. To see if a recent fact sheet has been published on scleroderma, simply go to the following hyperlink: **http://www.rarediseases.org/cgi-bin/nord/alphalist**. A complete guide on scleroderma can be purchased from NORD for a nominal fee.

Additional Web Sources

A number of Web sites that often link to government sites are available to the public. These can also point you in the direction of essential information. The following is a representative sample:

- AOL: **http://search.aol.com/cat.adp?id=168&layer=&from=subcats**

- drkoop.com®: **http://www.drkoop.com/conditions/ency/index.html**

- Family Village: **http://www.familyvillage.wisc.edu/specific.htm**

- Google: **http://directory.google.com/Top/Health/Conditions_and_Diseases/**

- Med Help International: **http://www.medhelp.org/HealthTopics/A.html**

- Open Directory Project: **http://dmoz.org/Health/Conditions_and_Diseases/**

- Yahoo.com: **http://dir.yahoo.com/Health/Diseases_and_Conditions/**

- WebMD®Health: **http://my.webmd.com/health_topics**

Vocabulary Builder

The material in this chapter may have contained a number of unfamiliar words. The following Vocabulary Builder introduces you to terms used in this chapter that have not been covered in the previous chapter:

Acetaminophen: Analgesic antipyretic derivative of acetanilide. It has weak anti-inflammatory properties and is used as a common analgesic, but may cause liver, blood cell, and kidney damage. [NIH]

Adjuvant: A substance which aids another, such as an auxiliary remedy; in immunology, nonspecific stimulator (e.g., BCG vaccine) of the immune response. [EU]

Ankle: That part of the lower limb directly above the foot. [NIH]

Antibiotic: A chemical substance produced by a microorganism which has the capacity, in dilute solutions, to inhibit the growth of or to kill other microorganisms. Antibiotics that are sufficiently nontoxic to the host are used as chemotherapeutic agents in the treatment of infectious diseases of man, animals and plants. [EU]

Antibody: An immunoglobulin molecule that has a specific amino acid sequence by virtue of which it interacts only with the antigen that induced its synthesis in cells of the lymphoid series (especially plasma cells), or with antigen closely related to it. Antibodies are classified according to their ode of action as agglutinins, bacteriolysins, haemolysins, opsonins, precipitins, etc. [EU]

Anxiety: The unpleasant emotional state consisting of psychophysiological responses to anticipation of unreal or imagined danger, ostensibly resulting from unrecognized intrapsychic conflict. Physiological concomitants include increased heart rate, altered respiration rate, sweating, trembling, weakness, and fatigue; psychological concomitants include feelings of impending danger, powerlessness, apprehension, and tension. [EU]

Arrhythmia: Any variation from the normal rhythm of the heart beat, including sinus arrhythmia, premature beat, heart block, atrial fibrillation, atrial flutter, pulsus alternans, and paroxysmal tachycardia. [EU]

Aspiration: The act of inhaling. [EU]

Autoimmunity: Process whereby the immune system reacts against the body's own tissues. Autoimmunity may produce or be caused by autoimmune diseases. [NIH]

Bacteria: Unicellular prokaryotic microorganisms which generally possess rigid cell walls, multiply by cell division, and exhibit three principal forms: round or coccal, rodlike or bacillary, and spiral or spirochetal. [NIH]

Baths: The immersion or washing of the body or any of its parts in water or other medium for cleansing or medical treatment. It includes bathing for personal hygiene as well as for medical purposes with the addition of therapeutic agents, such as alkalines, antiseptics, oil, etc. [NIH]

Biopsy: The removal and examination, usually microscopic, of tissue from the living body, performed to establish precise diagnosis. [EU]

Calcinosis: Pathologic deposition of calcium salts in tissues. [NIH]

Capillary: Any one of the minute vessels that connect the arterioles and venules, forming a network in nearly all parts of the body. Their walls act as semipermeable membranes for the interchange of various substances, including fluids, between the blood and tissue fluid; called also vas capillare. [EU]

Captopril: A potent and specific inhibitor of peptidyl-dipeptidase A. It blocks the conversion of angiotensin I to angiotensin II, a vasoconstrictor and important regulator of arterial blood pressure. Captopril acts to suppress the renin-angiotensin system and inhibits pressure responses to exogenous angiotensin. [NIH]

Carcinoma: A malignant new growth made up of epithelial cells tending to infiltrate the surrounding tissues and give rise to metastases. [EU]

Cardiomyopathy: A general diagnostic term designating primary myocardial disease, often of obscure or unknown etiology. [EU]

Caustic: An escharotic or corrosive agent. Called also cauterant. [EU]

Chronic: Persisting over a long period of time. [EU]

Collagen: The protein substance of the white fibres (collagenous fibres) of skin, tendon, bone, cartilage, and all other connective tissue; composed of molecules of tropocollagen (q.v.), it is converted into gelatin by boiling. collagenous pertaining to collagen; forming or producing collagen. [EU]

Constipation: Infrequent or difficult evacuation of the faeces. [EU]

Contracture: A condition of fixed high resistance to passive stretch of a muscle, resulting from fibrosis of the tissues supporting the muscles or the joints, or from disorders of the muscle fibres. [EU]

Cyclophosphamide: Precursor of an alkylating nitrogen mustard antineoplastic and immunosuppressive agent that must be activated in the liver to form the active aldophosphamide. It is used in the treatment of lymphomas, leukemias, etc. Its side effect, alopecia, has been made use of in defleecing sheep. Cyclophosphamide may also cause sterility, birth defects, mutations, and cancer. [NIH]

Degenerative: Undergoing degeneration : tending to degenerate; having the character of or involving degeneration; causing or tending to cause degeneration. [EU]

Dentists: Individuals licensed to practice dentistry. [NIH]

Dermatology: A medical specialty concerned with the skin, its structure, functions, diseases, and treatment. [NIH]

Diarrhea: Passage of excessively liquid or excessively frequent stools. [NIH]

Digestion: The process of breakdown of food for metabolism and use by the body. [NIH]

Enalapril: An angiotensin-converting enzyme inhibitor that is used to treat hypertension. [NIH]

Enzyme: A protein molecule that catalyses chemical reactions of other substances without itself being destroyed or altered upon completion of the reactions. Enzymes are classified according to the recommendations of the Nomenclature Committee of the International Union of Biochemistry. Each enzyme is assigned a recommended name and an Enzyme Commission (EC) number. They are divided into six main groups; oxidoreductases, transferases, hydrolases, lyases, isomerases, and ligases. [EU]

Erection: The condition of being made rigid and elevated; as erectile tissue when filled with blood. [EU]

Esophagitis: Inflammation, acute or chronic, of the esophagus caused by bacteria, chemicals, or trauma. [NIH]

Fatigue: The state of weariness following a period of exertion, mental or physical, characterized by a decreased capacity for work and reduced efficiency to respond to stimuli. [NIH]

Fibroblasts: Connective tissue cells which secrete an extracellular matrix rich in collagen and other macromolecules. [NIH]

Fibrosis: The formation of fibrous tissue; fibroid or fibrous degeneration [EU]

Gangrene: Death of tissue, usually in considerable mass and generally associated with loss of vascular (nutritive) supply and followed by bacterial invasion and putrefaction. [EU]

Gastrointestinal: Pertaining to or communicating with the stomach and intestine, as a gastrointestinal fistula. [EU]

Heartburn: Substernal pain or burning sensation, usually associated with regurgitation of gastric juice into the esophagus. [NIH]

Heredity: 1. the genetic transmission of a particular quality or trait from parent to offspring. 2. the genetic constitution of an individual. [EU]

Hormones: Chemical substances having a specific regulatory effect on the activity of a certain organ or organs. The term was originally applied to substances secreted by various endocrine glands and transported in the bloodstream to the target organs. It is sometimes extended to include those substances that are not produced by the endocrine glands but that have similar effects. [NIH]

Hypertension: Persistently high arterial blood pressure. Various criteria for its threshold have been suggested, ranging from 140 mm. Hg systolic and 90 mm. Hg diastolic to as high as 200 mm. Hg systolic and 110 mm. Hg diastolic. Hypertension may have no known cause (essential or idiopathic h.) or be associated with other primary diseases (secondary h.). [EU]

Idiopathic: Of the nature of an idiopathy; self-originated; of unknown causation. [EU]

Iloprost: An eicosanoid, derived from the cyclooxygenase pathway of arachidonic acid metabolism. It is a stable and synthetic analog of epoprostenol, but with a longer half-life than the parent compound. Its actions are similar to prostacyclin. Iloprost produces vasodilation and inhibits platelet aggregation. [NIH]

Inflammation: A pathological process characterized by injury or destruction of tissues caused by a variety of cytologic and chemical reactions. It is usually manifested by typical signs of pain, heat, redness, swelling, and loss of function. [NIH]

Intestines: The section of the alimentary canal from the stomach to the anus. It includes the large intestine and small intestine. [NIH]

Lesion: Any pathological or traumatic discontinuity of tissue or loss of function of a part. [EU]

Lip: Either of the two fleshy, full-blooded margins of the mouth. [NIH]

Lupus: A form of cutaneous tuberculosis. It is seen predominantly in women and typically involves the nasal, buccal, and conjunctival mucosa. [NIH]

Lymphoma: Any neoplastic disorder of the lymphoid tissue, the term lymphoma often is used alone to denote malignant lymphoma. [EU]

Malabsorption: Impaired intestinal absorption of nutrients. [EU]

Methotrexate: An antineoplastic antimetabolite with immunosuppressant properties. It is an inhibitor of dihydrofolate reductase and prevents the formation of tetrahydrofolate, necessary for synthesis of thymidylate, an essential component of DNA. [NIH]

Mobility: Capability of movement, of being moved, or of flowing freely. [EU]

Molecular: Of, pertaining to, or composed of molecules : a very small mass of matter. [EU]

Mycosis: Any disease caused by a fungus. [EU]

Myocarditis: Inflammation of the myocardium; inflammation of the muscular walls of the heart. [EU]

Myositis: Inflammation of a voluntary muscle. [EU]

Nausea: An unpleasant sensation, vaguely referred to the epigastrium and abdomen, and often culminating in vomiting. [EU]

Nifedipine: A potent vasodilator agent with calcium antagonistic action. It is a useful anti-anginal agent that also lowers blood pressure. The use of nifedipine as a tocolytic is being investigated. [NIH]

Oral: Pertaining to the mouth, taken through or applied in the mouth, as an oral medication or an oral thermometer. [EU]

Pilocarpine: A slowly hydrolyzed muscarinic agonist with no nicotinic effects. Pilocarpine is used as a miotic and in the treatment of glaucoma. [NIH]

Placenta: A highly vascular fetal organ through which the fetus absorbs oxygen and other nutrients and excretes carbon dioxide and other wastes. It begins to form about the eighth day of gestation when the blastocyst adheres to the DECIDUA. [NIH]

Pneumonia: Inflammation of the lungs with consolidation. [EU]

Porphyria: A pathological state in man and some lower animals that is often due to genetic factors, is characterized by abnormalities of porphyrin metabolism, and results in the excretion of large quantities of porphyrins in the urine and in extreme sensitivity to light. [EU]

Proteins: Polymers of amino acids linked by peptide bonds. The specific sequence of amino acids determines the shape and function of the protein. [NIH]

Pulmonary: Pertaining to the lungs. [EU]

Radiology: A specialty concerned with the use of x-ray and other forms of radiant energy in the diagnosis and treatment of disease. [NIH]

Rheumatoid: Resembling rheumatism. [EU]

Rheumatology: A subspecialty of internal medicine concerned with the study of inflammatory or degenerative processes and metabolic derangement of connective tissue structures which pertain to a variety of musculoskeletal disorders, such as arthritis. [NIH]

Sclerosis: A induration, or hardening; especially hardening of a part from inflammation and in diseases of the interstitial substance. The term is used chiefly for such a hardening of the nervous system due to hyperplasia of the connective tissue or to designate hardening of the blood vessels. [EU]

Soaps: Sodium or potassium salts of long chain fatty acids. These detergent substances are obtained by boiling natural oils or fats with caustic alkali. Sodium soaps are harder and are used as topical anti-infectives and vehicles in pills and liniments; potassium soaps are soft, used as vehicles for ointments and also as topical antimicrobials. [NIH]

Solvent: 1. dissolving; effecting a solution. 2. a liquid that dissolves or that is capable of dissolving; the component of a solution that is present in greater amount. [EU]

Stomach: An organ of digestion situated in the left upper quadrant of the abdomen between the termination of the esophagus and the beginning of the duodenum. [NIH]

Sweat: The fluid excreted by the sweat glands. It consists of water containing sodium chloride, phosphate, urea, ammonia, and other waste products. [NIH]

Systemic: Pertaining to or affecting the body as a whole. [EU]

Toxic: Pertaining to, due to, or of the nature of a poison or toxin; manifesting the symptoms of severe infection. [EU]

Transfusion: The introduction of whole blood or blood component directly into the blood stream. [EU]

Trichloroethylene: A highly volatile inhalation anesthetic used mainly in short surgical procedures where light anesthesia with good analgesia is required. It is also used as an industrial solvent. Prolonged exposure to high concentrations of the vapor can lead to cardiotoxicity and neurological impairment. [NIH]

Ulcer: A local defect, or excavation, of the surface of an organ or tissue; which is produced by the sloughing of inflammatory necrotic tissue. [EU]

Ulceration: 1. the formation or development of an ulcer. 2. an ulcer. [EU]

Vaccine: A suspension of attenuated or killed microorganisms (bacteria, viruses, or rickettsiae), administered for the prevention, amelioration or treatment of infectious diseases. [EU]

Vaginal: 1. of the nature of a sheath; ensheathing. 2. pertaining to the vagina. 3. pertaining to the tunica vaginalis testis. [EU]

Vascular: Pertaining to blood vessels or indicative of a copious blood supply. [EU]

Xerostomia: Dryness of the mouth from salivary gland dysfunction, as in Sjögren's syndrome. [EU]

CHAPTER 2. SEEKING GUIDANCE

Overview

Some patients are comforted by the knowledge that a number of organizations dedicate their resources to helping people with scleroderma. These associations can become invaluable sources of information and advice. Many associations offer aftercare support, financial assistance, and other important services. Furthermore, healthcare research has shown that support groups often help people to better cope with their conditions.[10] In addition to support groups, your physician can be a valuable source of guidance and support. Therefore, finding a physician that can work with your unique situation is a very important aspect of your care.

In this chapter, we direct you to resources that can help you find patient organizations and medical specialists. We begin by describing how to find associations and peer groups that can help you better understand and cope with scleroderma. The chapter ends with a discussion on how to find a doctor that is right for you.

Associations and Scleroderma

As mentioned by the Agency for Healthcare Research and Quality, sometimes the emotional side of an illness can be as taxing as the physical side.[11] You may have fears or feel overwhelmed by your situation. Everyone has different ways of dealing with disease or physical injury. Your attitude, your expectations, and how well you cope with your condition can all

---

[10] Churches, synagogues, and other houses of worship might also have groups that can offer you the social support you need.

[11] This section has been adapted from http://www.ahcpr.gov/consumer/diaginf5.htm.

influence your well-being. This is true for both minor conditions and serious illnesses. For example, a study on female breast cancer survivors revealed that women who participated in support groups lived longer and experienced better quality of life when compared with women who did not participate. In the support group, women learned coping skills and had the opportunity to share their feelings with other women in the same situation.

In addition to associations or groups that your doctor might recommend, we suggest that you consider the following list (if there is a fee for an association, you may want to check with your insurance provider to find out if the cost will be covered):

- **American Autoimmune Related Diseases Association, Inc**

  Address: American Autoimmune Related Diseases Association, Inc. Michigan National Bank Building, 15475 Gratiot Avenue, Detroit, MI 48205

  Telephone: (313) 371-8600 Toll-free: (800) 598- 4668

  Fax: (313) 371-6002

  Email: aarda@aol.com

  Web Site: http://www.aarda.org/

  Background: The American Autoimmune Related Diseases Association, Inc. (AARDA) is a national not-for-profit voluntary health agency dedicated to bringing a national focus to autoimmunity, a major cause of serious chronic diseases. The Association was founded for the purposes of supporting research to find a cure for autoimmune diseases and providing services to affected individuals. In addition, the Association's goals include increasing the public's awareness that autoimmunity is the cause of more than 80 serious chronic diseases; bringing national focus and collaborative effort among state and national voluntary health groups that represent autoimmune diseases; and serving as a national advocate for individuals and families affected by the physical, emotional, and financial effects of autoimmune disease. The American Autoimmune Related Diseases Association produces educational and support materials including fact sheets, brochures, pamphlets, and a newsletter entitled 'In Focus.'.

  Relevant area(s) of interest: Lupus, Psoriasis, Scleroderma, Vitiligo

- **Raynaud's and Scleroderma Association (UK)**

  Address: Raynaud's and Scleroderma Association (UK) 112 Crewe Road, Alsager, Cheshire, ST7 2JA, United Kingdom

  Telephone: 44 (0) 1270 872776 Toll-free: (800) 598- 4668

Fax: 44 (0) 1270 883556

Email: webmaster@raynauds.demon.co.uk

Web Site: http://www.raynauds.demon.co.uk

Background: The Raynaud's and Scleroderma Association (UK) is a voluntary, not- for-profit organization that was established in the United Kingdom in 1982. The Association is dedicated to promoting greater awareness of Raynaud's and scleroderma; offering support, information, and advice to affected individuals and family members; and assisting in the welfare of those who have disabilities resulting from or are chronically ill due to Raynaud's and scleroderma. Raynaud's is a condition characterized by sudden, episodic contraction of the blood vessels supplying the fingers and toes (digits), causing an interruption of blood flow to the digits. Symptoms and findings may include whitening of the digits due to lack of blood flow, eventual reddening of the digits as blood flow is gradually reestablished, and associated burning, tingling, and numbness. Episodes are usually triggered by exposure to cold temperatures. If the condition appears to occur spontaneously with no known cause, it is known as Raynaud's disease. When it occurs due to an underlying disorder, such as scleroderma or rheumatoid arthritis, the condition is referred to as Raynaud's phenomenon. Scleroderma is a rare disorder characterized by chronic thickening and hardening of the skin. The disorder may be localized, involving changes of the skin and underlying tissues (subcutaneous tissue and, in some cases, underlying muscle and bone), or may be systemic. In systemic scleroderma, there is thickening of the skin, abnormalities affecting blood vessels (e.g., seen in Raynaud's phenomenon), and degenerative (i.e., fibrotic) changes in various organs, such as the lungs, heart, and kidneys. The Raynaud's and Scleroderma Association (UK) is committed to providing information, support, and resources to affected individuals and family members and offering networking opportunities that enable individuals with the disorders to exchange ideas, information, and mutual support. In addition, the Association raises funds to further research into Raynaud's and scleroderma; disseminates the results of such research; and provides a listing of publications about the disorders. The Raynaud's and Scleroderma Association (UK) also has a web site on the Internet.

Relevant area(s) of interest: Scleroderma

- **Scleroderma Foundation, Inc**

  Address: Scleroderma Foundation, Inc. 89 Newbury Street, Suite 201, Danvers, MA 01923

  Telephone: (978) 750-4499 Toll-free: (800) 722-4673

Fax: (978) 750-9902

Email: sfinfo@scleroderma.org

Web Site: http://www.scleroderma.org

Background: The Scleroderma Foundation, Inc. (SF) is a not-for-profit organization dedicated to providing educational and emotional support for people with scleroderma and their families; increasing awareness of scleroderma; and supporting research to determine the disorder's cause, treatment, and cure. The Scleroderma Foundation testifies before Congress concerning the needs of people with scleroderma and works to increase public awareness through all forms of media. The organization raises research funding; institutes research grants; and conducts an annual conference. The Foundation also networks with other national health agencies on common concerns; assists people with scleroderma in securing Social Security and Disability benefits; and works with the medical community to promote better care and treatment.

Relevant area(s) of interest: Morphea, Scleroderma

- **Scleroderma Research Foundation**

  Address: Scleroderma Research Foundation 2320 Bath Street, Suite 315, Santa Barbara, CA 93105

  Telephone: (805) 563-9133 Toll-free: (800) 441-2873

  Fax: (805) 563-2402

  Email: srfcure@srfcure.org

  Web Site: http://www.srfcure.org

  Background: The Scleroderma Research Foundation is a voluntary research non-profit organization dedicated to finding a cure for Scleroderma by funding and facilitating ongoing medical research. The Foundation also seeks to increase public awareness and understanding of this disorder. Established in 1987, the Scleroderma Research Foundation created a team of scientific and biomedical advisors to identify and address key issues that may lead to a cure. The efforts of the Foundation and its advisory team have led to the opening of the Bay Area Scleroderma Research Center in San Francisco and the East Coast Scleroderma Research Center in Baltimore, both cross- institutional, multi-disciplinary research facilities. With participation of the National Institutes of Health (NIH) and several institutes and universities, the Foundation has also assisted in the creation of clinical laboratory tests that provide for the early diagnosis of several forms of Scleroderma. Moreover, with the assistance of the Foundation, significant progress has been achieved in the development of animal models for Scleroderma that may be a step toward development and evaluation of potential therapies. The Scleroderma Research Foundation has also been involved in the establishment of the importance of key cells that serve as catalysts in the onset of Scleroderma. The Scleroderma Research Foundation provides a variety of educational materials to affected individuals, family members, health care and research professionals, and the general public through its computer database, newsletters, articles, and video documentaries.

Relevant area(s) of interest: Morphea, Scleroderma

Finding More Associations

There are a number of directories that list additional medical associations that you may find useful. While not all of these directories will provide different information than what is listed above, by consulting all of them, you will have nearly exhausted all sources for patient associations.

The National Health Information Center (NHIC)

The National Health Information Center (NHIC) offers a free referral service to help people find organizations that provide information about scleroderma. For more information, see the NHIC's Web site at **http://www.health.gov/NHIC/** or contact an information specialist by calling 1-800-336-4797.

DIRLINE

A comprehensive source of information on associations is the DIRLINE database maintained by the National Library of Medicine. The database comprises some 10,000 records of organizations, research centers, and government institutes and associations which primarily focus on health and biomedicine. DIRLINE is available via the Internet at the following Web site: **http://dirline.nlm.nih.gov/**. Simply type in "scleroderma" (or a synonym) or the name of a topic, and the site will list information contained in the database on all relevant organizations.

The Combined Health Information Database

Another comprehensive source of information on healthcare associations is the Combined Health Information Database. Using the "Detailed Search" option, you will need to limit your search to "Organizations" and "scleroderma". Type the following hyperlink into your Web browser: **http://chid.nih.gov/detail/detail.html**. To find associations, use the drop boxes at the bottom of the search page where "You may refine your search by." For publication date, select "All Years." Then, select your preferred language and the format option "Organization Resource Sheet." By making these selections and typing in "scleroderma" (or synonyms) into the "For these words:" box, you will only receive results on organizations dealing with scleroderma. You should check back periodically with this database since it is updated every 3 months.

The National Organization for Rare Disorders, Inc.

The National Organization for Rare Disorders, Inc. has prepared a Web site that provides, at no charge, lists of associations organized by specific diseases. You can access this database at the following Web site: **http://www.rarediseases.org/cgi-bin/nord/searchpage**. Select the option called "Organizational Database (ODB)" and type "scleroderma" (or a synonym) in the search box.

Online Support Groups

In addition to support groups, commercial Internet service providers offer forums and chat rooms for people with different illnesses and conditions. WebMD®, for example, offers such a service at their Web site: **http://boards.webmd.com/roundtable**. These online self-help communities can help you connect with a network of people whose concerns are similar to yours. Online support groups are places where people can talk informally. If you read about a novel approach, consult with your doctor or other healthcare providers, as the treatments or discoveries you hear about may not be scientifically proven to be safe and effective.

Finding Doctors

One of the most important aspects of your treatment will be the relationship between you and your doctor or specialist. All patients with scleroderma must go through the process of selecting a physician. While this process will vary from person to person, the Agency for Healthcare Research and Quality makes a number of suggestions, including the following:[12]

- If you are in a managed care plan, check the plan's list of doctors first.

- Ask doctors or other health professionals who work with doctors, such as hospital nurses, for referrals.

- Call a hospital's doctor referral service, but keep in mind that these services usually refer you to doctors on staff at that particular hospital. The services do not have information on the quality of care that these doctors provide.

- Some local medical societies offer lists of member doctors. Again, these lists do not have information on the quality of care that these doctors provide.

Additional steps you can take to locate doctors include the following:

- Check with the associations listed earlier in this chapter.

- Information on doctors in some states is available on the Internet at **http://www.docboard.org**. This Web site is run by "Administrators in Medicine," a group of state medical board directors.

- The American Board of Medical Specialties can tell you if your doctor is board certified. "Certified" means that the doctor has completed a training program in a specialty and has passed an exam, or "board," to assess his or her knowledge, skills, and experience to provide quality patient care in that specialty. Primary care doctors may also be certified as specialists. The AMBS Web site is located at **http://www.abms.org/newsearch.asp**.[13] You can also contact the ABMS by phone at 1-866-ASK-ABMS.

- You can call the American Medical Association (AMA) at 800-665-2882 for information on training, specialties, and board certification for many licensed doctors in the United States. This information also can be found in "Physician Select" at the AMA's Web site: **http://www.ama-assn.org/aps/amahg.htm**.

If the previous sources did not meet your needs, you may want to log on to the Web site of the National Organization for Rare Disorders (NORD) at **http://www.rarediseases.org/**. NORD maintains a database of doctors with

---

[12] This section is adapted from the AHRQ: www.ahrq.gov/consumer/qntascii/qntdr.htm.
[13] While board certification is a good measure of a doctor's knowledge, it is possible to receive quality care from doctors who are not board certified.

expertise in various rare diseases. The Metabolic Information Network (MIN), 800-945-2188, also maintains a database of physicians with expertise in various metabolic diseases.

Finding a Dermatologist

To find a dermatologist in your area, you can use the "Find a Dermatologist" search engine provided by the American Academy of Dermatology. With a membership of 13,000, the American Academy of Dermatology represents virtually all practicing dermatologists in the United States and Canada. Type the following Web address into your browser to begin your search: **http://www.aad.org/DermSearch/index.html**. To search for dermatologists by U.S. state, enter your state into the search box and click "Search." To search for dermatologists practicing outside the U.S., select "international members." Enter your country and click the "Search" button.

Selecting Your Doctor[14]

When you have compiled a list of prospective doctors, call each of their offices. First, ask if the doctor accepts your health insurance plan and if he or she is taking new patients. If the doctor is not covered by your plan, ask yourself if you are prepared to pay the extra costs. The next step is to schedule a visit with your chosen physician. During the first visit you will have the opportunity to evaluate your doctor and to find out if you feel comfortable with him or her. Ask yourself, did the doctor:

- Give me a chance to ask questions about scleroderma?
- Really listen to my questions?
- Answer in terms I understood?
- Show respect for me?
- Ask me questions?
- Make me feel comfortable?
- Address the health problem(s) I came with?
- Ask me my preferences about different kinds of treatments for scleroderma?

---

[14] This section has been adapted from the AHRQ: www.ahrq.gov/consumer/qntascii/qntdr.htm.

- Spend enough time with me?

Trust your instincts when deciding if the doctor is right for you. But remember, it might take time for the relationship to develop. It takes more than one visit for you and your doctor to get to know each other.

Working with Your Doctor[15]

Research has shown that patients who have good relationships with their doctors tend to be more satisfied with their care and have better results. Here are some tips to help you and your doctor become partners:

- You know important things about your symptoms and your health history. Tell your doctor what you think he or she needs to know.

- It is important to tell your doctor personal information, even if it makes you feel embarrassed or uncomfortable.

- Bring a "health history" list with you (and keep it up to date).

- Always bring any medications you are currently taking with you to the appointment, or you can bring a list of your medications including dosage and frequency information. Talk about any allergies or reactions you have had to your medications.

- Tell your doctor about any natural or alternative medicines you are taking.

- Bring other medical information, such as x-ray films, test results, and medical records.

- Ask questions. If you don't, your doctor will assume that you understood everything that was said.

- Write down your questions before your visit. List the most important ones first to make sure that they are addressed.

- Consider bringing a friend with you to the appointment to help you ask questions. This person can also help you understand and/or remember the answers.

- Ask your doctor to draw pictures if you think that this would help you understand.

- Take notes. Some doctors do not mind if you bring a tape recorder to help you remember things, but always ask first.

---

15 This section has been adapted from the AHRQ:
www.ahrq.gov/consumer/qntascii/qntdr.htm.

- Let your doctor know if you need more time. If there is not time that day, perhaps you can speak to a nurse or physician assistant on staff or schedule a telephone appointment.

- Take information home. Ask for written instructions. Your doctor may also have brochures and audio and videotapes that can help you.

- After leaving the doctor's office, take responsibility for your care. If you have questions, call. If your symptoms get worse or if you have problems with your medication, call. If you had tests and do not hear from your doctor, call for your test results. If your doctor recommended that you have certain tests, schedule an appointment to get them done. If your doctor said you should see an additional specialist, make an appointment.

By following these steps, you will enhance the relationship you will have with your physician.

Broader Health-Related Resources

In addition to the references above, the NIH has set up guidance Web sites that can help patients find healthcare professionals. These include:[16]

- Caregivers:
  http://www.nlm.nih.gov/medlineplus/caregivers.html

- Choosing a Doctor or Healthcare Service:
  http://www.nlm.nih.gov/medlineplus/choosingadoctororhealthcareserv ice.html

- Hospitals and Health Facilities:
  http://www.nlm.nih.gov/medlineplus/healthfacilities.html

Vocabulary Builder

The following vocabulary builder provides definitions of words used in this chapter that have not been defined in previous chapters:

Keratoconjunctivitis: Inflammation of the cornea and conjunctiva. [EU]

Lacrimal: Pertaining to the tears. [EU]

---

[16] You can access this information at:
http://www.nlm.nih.gov/medlineplus/healthsystem.html.

Psoriasis: A common genetically determined, chronic, inflammatory skin disease characterized by rounded erythematous, dry, scaling patches. The lesions have a predilection for nails, scalp, genitalia, extensor surfaces, and the lumbosacral region. Accelerated epidermopoiesis is considered to be the fundamental pathologic feature in psoriasis. [NIH]

Vitiligo: A disorder consisting of areas of macular depigmentation, commonly on extensor aspects of extremities, on the face or neck, and in skin folds. Age of onset is often in young adulthood and the condition tends to progress gradually with lesions enlarging and extending until a quiescent state is reached. [NIH]

CHAPTER 3. CLINICAL TRIALS AND SCLERODERMA

Overview

Very few medical conditions have a single treatment. The basic treatment guidelines that your physician has discussed with you, or those that you have found using the techniques discussed in Chapter 1, may provide you with all that you will require. For some patients, current treatments can be enhanced with new or innovative techniques currently under investigation. In this chapter, we will describe how clinical trials work and show you how to keep informed of trials concerning scleroderma.

What Is a Clinical Trial?[17]

Clinical trials involve the participation of people in medical research. Most medical research begins with studies in test tubes and on animals. Treatments that show promise in these early studies may then be tried with people. The only sure way to find out whether a new treatment is safe, effective, and better than other treatments for scleroderma is to try it on patients in a clinical trial.

---

[17] The discussion in this chapter has been adapted from the NIH and the NEI: www.nei.nih.gov/netrials/ctivr.htm.

What Kinds of Clinical Trials Are There?

Clinical trials are carried out in three phases:

- **Phase I.** Researchers first conduct Phase I trials with small numbers of patients and healthy volunteers. If the new treatment is a medication, researchers also try to determine how much of it can be given safely.

- **Phase II.** Researchers conduct Phase II trials in small numbers of patients to find out the effect of a new treatment on scleroderma.

- **Phase III.** Finally, researchers conduct Phase III trials to find out how new treatments for scleroderma compare with standard treatments already being used. Phase III trials also help to determine if new treatments have any side effects. These trials--which may involve hundreds, perhaps thousands, of people--can also compare new treatments with no treatment.

How Is a Clinical Trial Conducted?

Various organizations support clinical trials at medical centers, hospitals, universities, and doctors' offices across the United States. The "principal investigator" is the researcher in charge of the study at each facility participating in the clinical trial. Most clinical trial researchers are medical doctors, academic researchers, and specialists. The "clinic coordinator" knows all about how the study works and makes all the arrangements for your visits.

All doctors and researchers who take part in the study on scleroderma carefully follow a detailed treatment plan called a protocol. This plan fully explains how the doctors will treat you in the study. The "protocol" ensures that all patients are treated in the same way, no matter where they receive care.

Clinical trials are controlled. This means that researchers compare the effects of the new treatment with those of the standard treatment. In some cases, when no standard treatment exists, the new treatment is compared with no treatment. Patients who receive the new treatment are in the treatment group. Patients who receive a standard treatment or no treatment are in the "control" group. In some clinical trials, patients in the treatment group get a new medication while those in the control group get a placebo. A placebo is a harmless substance, a "dummy" pill, that has no effect on scleroderma. In other clinical trials, where a new surgery or device (not a medicine) is being tested, patients in the control group may receive a "sham treatment." This treatment, like a placebo, has no effect on scleroderma and does not harm patients.

Researchers assign patients "randomly" to the treatment or control group. This is like flipping a coin to decide which patients are in each group. If you choose to participate in a clinical trial, you will not know which group you will be appointed to. The chance of any patient getting the new treatment is about 50 percent. You cannot request to receive the new treatment instead of the placebo or sham treatment. Often, you will not know until the study is over whether you have been in the treatment group or the control group. This is called a "masked" study. In some trials, neither doctors nor patients know who is getting which treatment. This is called a "double masked" study. These types of trials help to ensure that the perceptions of the patients or doctors will not affect the study results.

Natural History Studies

Unlike clinical trials in which patient volunteers may receive new treatments, natural history studies provide important information to researchers on how scleroderma develops over time. A natural history study follows patient volunteers to see how factors such as age, sex, race, or family history might make some people more or less at risk for scleroderma. A natural history study may also tell researchers if diet, lifestyle, or occupation affects how a disease or disorder develops and progresses. Results from these studies provide information that helps answer questions such as: How fast will a disease or disorder usually progress? How bad will the condition become? Will treatment be needed?

What Is Expected of Patients in a Clinical Trial?

Not everyone can take part in a clinical trial for a specific disease or disorder. Each study enrolls patients with certain features or eligibility criteria. These criteria may include the type and stage of disease or disorder, as well as, the age and previous treatment history of the patient. You or your doctor can contact the sponsoring organization to find out more about specific clinical trials and their eligibility criteria. If you are interested in joining a clinical trial, your doctor must contact one of the trial's investigators and provide details about your diagnosis and medical history.

If you participate in a clinical trial, you may be required to have a number of medical tests. You may also need to take medications and/or undergo surgery. Depending upon the treatment and the examination procedure, you may be required to receive inpatient hospital care. Or, you may have to return to the medical facility for follow-up examinations. These exams help find out how well the treatment is working. Follow-up studies can take months or years. However, the success of the clinical trial often depends on learning what happens to patients over a long period of time. Only patients who continue to return for follow-up examinations can provide this important long-term information.

Recent Trials on Scleroderma

The National Institutes of Health and other organizations sponsor trials on various diseases and disorders. Because funding for research goes to the medical areas that show promising research opportunities, it is not possible for the NIH or others to sponsor clinical trials for every disease and disorder at all times. The following lists recent trials dedicated to scleroderma.[18] If the trial listed by the NIH is still recruiting, you may be eligible. If it is no longer recruiting or has been completed, then you can contact the sponsors to learn more about the study and, if published, the results. Further information on the trial is available at the Web site indicated. Please note that some trials may no longer be recruiting patients or are otherwise closed. Before contacting sponsors of a clinical trial, consult with your physician who can help you determine if you might benefit from participation.

- **Autologous Stem Cell Transplant For Systemic Sclerosis**

  Condition(s): Scleroderma, Systemic

  Study Status: This study is currently recruiting patients.

  Sponsor(s): National Institute of Arthritis and Musculoskeletal and Skin Diseases (NIAMS); University of Pittsburgh Cancer Institute; Amgen; Sangstat Medical Corporation

  Purpose - Excerpt: Patients with systemic sclerosis undergo tests,sign informed consent. Patients are admitted to hospital for a day of chemotherapy. Patients go home and receive a shot of G-CSF for about 10 days, then a procedure called Leukapheresis begins and is done as outpatient for up to 4 days. Chemotherapy is given for 5 days. The doses of chemotherapy will be increased after every three patients if there are no serious side effects. Thymoglobulin, an immunosuppressing drug, will be given for 3 days. On day 0 patient receive infusion of stem cells. It will take 2-4 weeks to recover from side effects of this treatment. Patient Involvement:Patients must be stay in the Pittsburgh area for their

---

18 These are listed at www.ClinicalTrials.gov.

treatment, are required to use appropriate birth control to prevent pregnancy.Patients will have blood sample 16 times during first 2 years of treatment and return to Pittsburgh 12, 18, and 24 months after the transplant to be evaluated and to give blood samples.

Phase(s): Phase I

Study Type: Interventional

Contact(s): see Web site below

Web Site:
http://clinicaltrials.gov/ct/gui/show/NCT00040651;jsessionid=D254F5 91722154486524094046D74125

- **Oral Type I Collagen in Scleroderma**

  Condition(s): Scleroderma

  Study Status: This study is currently recruiting patients.

  Sponsor(s): National Institute of Arthritis and Musculoskeletal and Skin Diseases (NIAMS)

  Purpose - Excerpt: This is a 15-month study to find out if taking type I collagen by mouth will improve diffuse systemic sclerosis (scleroderma). We will randomly assign 168 patients to receive type I collagen from cows or a placebo (inactive treatment) for 12 months. We will examine patients and do laboratory tests once every 4 months during the 12-month treatment period and once more at 15 months.

  Phase(s): Phase II

  Study Type: Interventional

  Contact(s): see Web site below

  Web Site:
  http://clinicaltrials.gov/ct/gui/show/NCT00005675;jsessionid=D254F5 91722154486524094046D74125

- **Psychological Treatments for Scleroderma**

  Condition(s): Pain; Depression; Scleroderma; Systemic Sclerosis

  Study Status: This study is currently recruiting patients.

  Sponsor(s): National Institute of Arthritis and Musculoskeletal and Skin Diseases (NIAMS)

  Purpose - Excerpt: This study will examine the effectiveness of two psychological treatment approaches designed to help people who have scleroderma with three important areas of daily living: pain, depression, and distress about changes in appearance. We will also study the impact of depression on the psychological treatments. Because psychological approaches requiring a trained professional can be expensive and are often not available to most patients, we will also look at the effectiveness of a self-help treatment approach.

Phase(s): Phase II

Study Type: Interventional

Contact(s): Jennifer A. Haythornthwaite 410-614-9850 jhaythor@jhmi.edu; Maryland; Johns Hopkins Bayview Medical Center, Baltimore, Maryland, United States; Recruiting; Keya Medley 410-614-3396 1. Study chairs or principal investigators: Jennifer A. Haythornthwaite, Principal Investigator; Johns Hopkins University

Web Site:
http://clinicaltrials.gov/ct/gui/show/NCT00007267;jsessionid=D254F5 91722154486524094046D74125

- **Scleroderma Lung Study**

  Condition(s): Lung Diseases; Pulmonary Fibrosis; Systemic Scleroderma; Scleroderma, systemic

  Study Status: This study is currently recruiting patients.

  Sponsor(s): National Heart, Lung, and Blood Institute (NHLBI)

  Purpose - Excerpt: To evaluate the efficacy and safety of cyclophosphamide versus placebo for the prevention and progression of symptomatic pulmonary disease in patients with systemic sclerosis.

  Phase(s): Phase III

  Study Type: Treatment, Prevention

  Contact(s): see Web site below

  Web Site:
  http://clinicaltrials.gov/ct/gui/show/NCT00004563;jsessionid=D254F5 91722154486524094046D74125

- **Six month clinical research study for patients with moderate or severe dry eye syndrome**

  Condition(s): Keratoconjunctivitis Sicca; Sjogren's Syndrome; Lupus Erythematosus, Systemic; Arthritis, Rheumatoid; Scleroderma, Systemic

  Study Status: This study is currently recruiting patients.

  Sponsor(s): Allergan

  Purpose - Excerpt: A six-month clinical research trial to evaluate the effectiveness of an investigational medication for the treatment of dry eye syndrome in patients that have been diagnosed with moderate to severe dry eye syndrome, an autoimmune disorder AND/OR females 65 years of age or older.

Phase(s): Phase III

Study Type: Interventional

Contact(s): see Web site below

Web Site:
http://clinicaltrials.gov/ct/gui/show/NCT00025818;jsessionid=D254F5 91722154486524094046D74125

- **Idiopathic Pulmonary Fibrosis--Pathogenesis and Staging - SCOR in Occupational and Immunological Lung Diseases**

  Condition(s): Lung Diseases; Pulmonary Fibrosis; Lung diseases, interstitial; Scleroderma, systemic

  Study Status: This study is completed.

  Sponsor(s): National Heart, Lung, and Blood Institute (NHLBI)

  Purpose - Excerpt: To conduct cross-sectional and longitudinal studies of patients with idiopathic pulmonary fibrosis (IPF) and patients with progressive systemic sclerosis (PSS), with and without associated lung disease.

  Study Type: Longitudinal Human Study

  Contact(s): see Web site below

  Web Site:
  http://clinicaltrials.gov/ct/gui/show/NCT00005317;jsessionid=D254F5 91722154486524094046D74125

- **Phase II Study of Recombinant Relaxin for Progressive Systemic Sclerosis**

  Condition(s): Systemic Sclerosis

  Study Status: This study is completed.

  Sponsor(s): National Center for Research Resources (NCRR); National Institute of Arthritis and Musculoskeletal and Skin Diseases (NIAMS); Stanford University

  Purpose - Excerpt: Objectives: I. Determine whether parenteral relaxin improves skin tightness, Raynaud's phenomenon, digital morbidity, and digital ulcers in a patient with progressive systemic sclerosis (scleroderma). II. Determine whether relaxin decreases collagen production by fibroblasts in vivo and cultured from skin biopsies.

Phase(s): Phase II

Study Type: Interventional

Contact(s):. Study chairs or principal investigators: G. Scott Herron, Study Chair; Stanford University

Web Site:
http://clinicaltrials.gov/ct/gui/show/NCT00004380;jsessionid=D254F5 91722154486524094046D74125

Benefits and Risks[19]

What Are the Benefits of Participating in a Clinical Trial?

If you are interested in a clinical trial, it is important to realize that your participation can bring many benefits to you and society at large:

- A new treatment could be more effective than the current treatment for scleroderma. Although only half of the participants in a clinical trial receive the experimental treatment, if the new treatment is proved to be more effective and safer than the current treatment, then those patients who did not receive the new treatment during the clinical trial may be among the first to benefit from it when the study is over.

- If the treatment is effective, then it may improve health or prevent diseases or disorders.

- Clinical trial patients receive the highest quality of medical care. Experts watch them closely during the study and may continue to follow them after the study is over.

- People who take part in trials contribute to scientific discoveries that may help other people with scleroderma. In cases where certain diseases or disorders run in families, your participation may lead to better care or prevention for your family members.

---

[19] This section has been adapted from ClinicalTrials.gov, a service of the National Institutes of Health:
http://www.clinicaltrials.gov/ct/gui/c/a1r/info/whatis?JServSessionIdzone_ct=9jmun6f2 91.

The Informed Consent

Once you agree to take part in a clinical trial, you will be asked to sign an "informed consent." This document explains a clinical trial's risks and benefits, the researcher's expectations of you, and your rights as a patient.

What Are the Risks?

Clinical trials may involve risks as well as benefits. Whether or not a new treatment will work cannot be known ahead of time. There is always a chance that a new treatment may not work better than a standard treatment. There is also the possibility that it may be harmful. The treatment you receive may cause side effects that are serious enough to require medical attention.

How Is Patient Safety Protected?

Clinical trials can raise fears of the unknown. Understanding the safeguards that protect patients can ease some of these fears. Before a clinical trial begins, researchers must get approval from their hospital's Institutional Review Board (IRB), an advisory group that makes sure a clinical trial is designed to protect patient safety. During a clinical trial, doctors will closely watch you to see if the treatment is working and if you are experiencing any side effects. All the results are carefully recorded and reviewed. In many cases, experts from the Data and Safety Monitoring Committee carefully monitor each clinical trial and can recommend that a study be stopped at any time. You will only be asked to take part in a clinical trial as a volunteer giving informed consent.

What Are a Patient's Rights in a Clinical Trial?

If you are eligible for a clinical trial, you will be given information to help you decide whether or not you want to participate. As a patient, you have the right to:

- Information on all known risks and benefits of the treatments in the study.

- Know how the researchers plan to carry out the study, for how long, and where.

- Know what is expected of you.

- Know any costs involved for you or your insurance provider.

- Know before any of your medical or personal information is shared with other researchers involved in the clinical trial.

- Talk openly with doctors and ask any questions.

After you join a clinical trial, you have the right to:

- Leave the study at any time. Participation is strictly voluntary. However, you should not enroll if you do not plan to complete the study.

- Receive any new information about the new treatment.

- Continue to ask questions and get answers.

- Maintain your privacy. Your name will not appear in any reports based on the study.

- Know whether you participated in the treatment group or the control group (once the study has been completed).

What about Costs?

In some clinical trials, the research facility pays for treatment costs and other associated expenses. You or your insurance provider may have to pay for costs that are considered standard care. These things may include inpatient hospital care, laboratory and other tests, and medical procedures. You also may need to pay for travel between your home and the clinic. You should find out about costs before committing to participation in the trial. If you have health insurance, find out exactly what it will cover. If you don't have health insurance, or if your insurance company will not cover your costs, talk to the clinic staff about other options for covering the cost of your care.

What Should You Ask before Deciding to Join a Clinical Trial?

Questions you should ask when thinking about joining a clinical trial include the following:

- What is the purpose of the clinical trial?

- What are the standard treatments for scleroderma? Why do researchers think the new treatment may be better? What is likely to happen to me with or without the new treatment?

- What tests and treatments will I need? Will I need surgery? Medication? Hospitalization?

- How long will the treatment last? How often will I have to come back for follow-up exams?

- What are the treatment's possible benefits to my condition? What are the short- and long-term risks? What are the possible side effects?

- Will the treatment be uncomfortable? Will it make me feel sick? If so, for how long?

- How will my health be monitored?

- Where will I need to go for the clinical trial? How will I get there?

- How much will it cost to be in the study? What costs are covered by the study? How much will my health insurance cover?

- Will I be able to see my own doctor? Who will be in charge of my care?

- Will taking part in the study affect my daily life? Do I have time to participate?

- How do I feel about taking part in a clinical trial? Are there family members or friends who may benefit from my contributions to new medical knowledge?

Keeping Current on Clinical Trials

Various government agencies maintain databases on trials. The U.S. National Institutes of Health, through the National Library of Medicine, has developed ClinicalTrials.gov to provide patients, family members, and physicians with current information about clinical research across the broadest number of diseases and conditions.

The site was launched in February 2000 and currently contains approximately 5,700 clinical studies in over 59,000 locations worldwide, with most studies being conducted in the United States. ClinicalTrials.gov receives about 2 million hits per month and hosts approximately 5,400 visitors daily. To access this database, simply go to their Web site (**www.clinicaltrials.gov**) and search by "scleroderma" (or synonyms).

While ClinicalTrials.gov is the most comprehensive listing of NIH-supported clinical trials available, not all trials are in the database. The database is updated regularly, so clinical trials are continually being added. The following is a list of specialty databases affiliated with the National Institutes of Health that offer additional information on trials:

- For clinical studies at the Warren Grant Magnuson Clinical Center located in Bethesda, Maryland, visit their Web site: **http://clinicalstudies.info.nih.gov/**

- For clinical studies conducted at the Bayview Campus in Baltimore, Maryland, visit their Web site: **http://www.jhbmc.jhu.edu/studies/index.html**

General References

The following references describe clinical trials and experimental medical research. They have been selected to ensure that they are likely to be available from your local or online bookseller or university medical library. These references are usually written for healthcare professionals, so you may consider consulting with a librarian or bookseller who might recommend a particular reference. The following includes some of the most readily available references (sorted alphabetically by title; hyperlinks provide rankings, information and reviews at Amazon.com):

- **A Guide to Patient Recruitment : Today's Best Practices & Proven Strategies** by Diana L. Anderson; Paperback - 350 pages (2001), CenterWatch, Inc.; ISBN: 1930624115; **http://www.amazon.com/exec/obidos/ASIN/1930624115/icongroupinterna**

- **A Step-By-Step Guide to Clinical Trials** by Marilyn Mulay, R.N., M.S., OCN; Spiral-bound - 143 pages Spiral edition (2001), Jones & Bartlett Pub; ISBN: 0763715697; **http://www.amazon.com/exec/obidos/ASIN/0763715697/icongroupinterna**

- **The CenterWatch Directory of Drugs in Clinical Trials** by CenterWatch; Paperback - 656 pages (2000), CenterWatch, Inc.; ISBN: 0967302935; **http://www.amazon.com/exec/obidos/ASIN/0967302935/icongroupinterna**

- **The Complete Guide to Informed Consent in Clinical Trials** by Terry Hartnett (Editor); Paperback - 164 pages (2000), PharmSource Information Services, Inc.; ISBN: 0970153309; **http://www.amazon.com/exec/obidos/ASIN/0970153309/icongroupinterna**

- **Dictionary for Clinical Trials** by Simon Day; Paperback - 228 pages (1999), John Wiley & Sons; ISBN: 0471985961; http://www.amazon.com/exec/obidos/ASIN/0471985961/icongroupinterna

- **Extending Medicare Reimbursement in Clinical Trials** by Institute of Medicine Staff (Editor), et al; Paperback 1st edition (2000), National Academy Press; ISBN: 0309068886; http://www.amazon.com/exec/obidos/ASIN/0309068886/icongroupinterna

- **Handbook of Clinical Trials** by Marcus Flather (Editor); Paperback (2001), Remedica Pub Ltd; ISBN: 1901346293; http://www.amazon.com/exec/obidos/ASIN/1901346293/icongroupinterna

Vocabulary Builder

The following vocabulary builder gives definitions of words used in this chapter that have not been defined in previous chapters:

Chemotherapy: The treatment of disease by means of chemicals that have a specific toxic effect upon the disease - producing microorganisms or that selectively destroy cancerous tissue. [EU]

Homologous: Corresponding in structure, position, origin, etc., as (a) the feathers of a bird and the scales of a fish, (b) antigen and its specific antibody, (c) allelic chromosomes. [EU]

Infusion: The therapeutic introduction of a fluid other than blood, as saline solution, solution, into a vein. [EU]

Interstitial: Pertaining to or situated between parts or in the interspaces of a tissue. [EU]

Leukapheresis: The preparation of leukocyte concentrates with the return of red cells and leukocyte-poor plasma to the donor. [NIH]

Parenteral: Not through the alimentary canal but rather by injection through some other route, as subcutaneous, intramuscular, intraorbital, intracapsular, intraspinal, intrasternal, intravenous, etc. [EU]

Predisposition: A latent susceptibility to disease which may be activated under certain conditions, as by stress. [EU]

Progressive: Advancing; going forward; going from bad to worse; increasing in scope or severity. [EU]

Recombinant: 1. a cell or an individual with a new combination of genes not found together in either parent; usually applied to linked genes. [EU]

Reconstitution: 1. a type of regeneration in which a new organ forms by the rearrangement of tissues rather than from new formation at an injured surface. 2. the restoration to original form of a substance previously altered for preservation and storage, as the restoration to a liquid state of blood serum or plasma that has been dried and stored. [EU]

Refractory: Not readily yielding to treatment. [EU]

Symptomatic: 1. pertaining to or of the nature of a symptom. 2. indicative (of a particular disease or disorder). 3. exhibiting the symptoms of a particular disease but having a different cause. 4. directed at the allying of symptoms, as symptomatic treatment. [EU]

Toxicity: The quality of being poisonous, especially the degree of virulence of a toxic microbe or of a poison. [EU]

Transplantation: The grafting of tissues taken from the patient's own body or from another. [EU]

PART II: ADDITIONAL RESOURCES AND ADVANCED MATERIAL

ABOUT PART II

In Part II, we introduce you to additional resources and advanced research on scleroderma. All too often, patients who conduct their own research are overwhelmed by the difficulty in finding and organizing information. The purpose of the following chapters is to provide you an organized and structured format to help you find additional information resources on scleroderma. In Part II, as in Part I, our objective is not to interpret the latest advances on scleroderma or render an opinion. Rather, our goal is to give you access to original research and to increase your awareness of sources you may not have already considered. In this way, you will come across the advanced materials often referred to in pamphlets, books, or other general works. Once again, some of this material is technical in nature, so consultation with a professional familiar with scleroderma is suggested.

CHAPTER 4. STUDIES ON SCLERODERMA

Overview

Every year, academic studies are published on scleroderma or related conditions. Broadly speaking, there are two types of studies. The first are peer reviewed. Generally, the content of these studies has been reviewed by scientists or physicians. Peer-reviewed studies are typically published in scientific journals and are usually available at medical libraries. The second type of studies is non-peer reviewed. These works include summary articles that do not use or report scientific results. These often appear in the popular press, newsletters, or similar periodicals.

In this chapter, we will show you how to locate peer-reviewed references and studies on scleroderma. We will begin by discussing research that has been summarized and is free to view by the public via the Internet. We then show you how to generate a bibliography on scleroderma and teach you how to keep current on new studies as they are published or undertaken by the scientific community.

The Combined Health Information Database

The Combined Health Information Database summarizes studies across numerous federal agencies. To limit your investigation to research studies and scleroderma, you will need to use the advanced search options. First, go to **http://chid.nih.gov/index.html**. From there, select the "Detailed Search" option (or go directly to that page with the following hyperlink: **http://chid.nih.gov/detail/detail.html**). The trick in extracting studies is found in the drop boxes at the bottom of the search page where "You may refine your search by." Select the dates and language you prefer, and the format option "Journal Article." At the top of the search form, select the number of records you would like to see (we recommend 100) and check the box to display "whole records." We recommend that you type in "scleroderma" (or synonyms) into the "For these words:" box. Consider using the option "anywhere in record" to make your search as broad as possible. If you want to limit the search to only a particular field, such as the title of the journal, then select this option in the "Search in these fields" drop box. The following is a sample of what you can expect from this type of search:

- **Gastrointestinal Manifestations of Scleroderma**

  Source: Gastroenterology Clinics of North America. 27(3): 563-594. September 1998.

  Summary: This journal article provides health professionals with information on the pathophysiology, clinical presentation, management, and complications of the gastrointestinal manifestations common in scleroderma. Gastrointestinal problems may be the presenting symptoms for the diagnosis and may precede the actual diagnosis by months or years. The esophagus is the most frequently affected, but functional problems of the anorectum, small bowel, colon, and stomach may also occur. The pathophysiologic mechanism appears to be smooth muscle atrophy and, to a lesser degree, fibrosis. These changes result in gastrointestinal motility disturbances and may cause gastroesophageal reflux disease (GERD), pseudo-obstruction, bacterial overgrowth, and defecatory disorders. Malnutrition may be a serious consequence. Approaches to treating GERD include behavioral modification, medical therapy, and surgical intervention. Gastric and intestinal disorders associated with scleroderma may be treated with promotility drugs, bowel rest and decompression, and antibiotic therapy. Methods of treating colonic and anorectal disorders in scleroderma patients include increasing fluids and dietary intake of fiber, instituting a low-residue diet, and using antidiarrheal agents. Evaluating a particular symptom in a patient who has scleroderma may lead to treatment strategies that improve well-being and quality of life. 4 figures, 3 tables, and 137 references. (Sum-M).

- **Management of Localized Scleroderma**

  Source: Seminars in Cutaneous Medicine and Surgery. 17(1): 34-40. March 1998.

  Summary: This journal article provides health professionals with information on the pathogenesis and treatment of localized scleroderma, which denotes a spectrum of conditions characterized by circumscribed fibrotic areas involving different levels of the dermis, subcutis, and sometimes underlying soft tissue and bone. Different clinical manifestations of localized scleroderma exist. From a therapeutic viewpoint, a subdivision that includes the extent and level of fibrosis in the skin, resulting in plaque, generalized, linear, and deep type, is helpful in choosing the appropriate therapy and determining its effectiveness. Although the pathogenesis of the different types of localized scleroderma is unknown, the pathological conditions observed in patients who have it affect mainly the connective tissue; however, this is associated with alterations of the immunologic system and the vessel walls. Although the clinical course of the disease is often benign, widespread lesions and disabling joint contractures may lead to significant complications. Numerous therapeutic agents have been reported to be effective in this disease spectrum; they include topical steroid creams; oral medications such as vitamins E and D3, phenytoin, retinoids, antibiotics, griseofulvin, interferon gamma, and oral steroids; ultraviolet A (UVA) irradiation and psoralen UVA therapy; physical therapy; and surgery. 2 figures, 2 tables, and 54 references. (AA-M).

- **Managing Skin Lesions of Scleroderma a Challenge**

  Source: Journal of Musculoskeletal Medicine. 12,15; November 1995.

  Summary: This journal article for health professionals answer questions about treating lesions associated with scleroderma and managing generalized scleroderma . Studies on the management of generalized scleroderma are recommended. Evidence for and against various treatments to ameliorate the skin manifestations of scleroderma is reviewed, focusing on results of trials of D- penicillamine (DPA), extracorporeal photopheresis , and immunosuppressive therapy. In addition, recommendations for using DPA are provided, and adverse effects of DPA are identified. 8 references.

- **Scleroderma: Not One of the Usual Suspects**

  Source: Advance for Speech-Language Pathologists and Audiologists. 7(1): 11, 42. January 7, 1997.

  Contact: Available from Merion Publications, Inc. 650 Park Avenue, Box 61556, King of Prussia, PA 19406-0956. (800) 355-1088 or (610) 265-7812.

  Summary: This article, from a professional newsletter for speech language pathologists and audiologists, reviews the condition of scleroderma. Scleroderma is a rare autoimmune disease characterized by fibrosis of the skin and internal organs; the disease can affect the mouth, vocal cords, and larynx. The article interviews two clinicians. Topics include the speech problems associated with scleroderma; the effect of collagen infiltration in the vocal cords; Sjogren's syndrome; scleroderma treatment programs; swallowing impairments that may accompany scleroderma; risk factors for cancer in the oral cavity, vocal cords, and larynx; patient assessment considerations; staging of disease; and intervention options, ranging from conservative to aggressive treatments. The article concludes with a brief discussion of the importance of increasing physician and public awareness of scleroderma. The contact information for the two clinicians interviewed is provided. 2 figures.

- **Connective Tissue Disease Update: Focus on Scleroderma**

  Source: Consultant. 39(7): 2071-2074,2077-2078,2081-2082. July 1999.

  Summary: This journal article, the second in a three-part series on connective tissue diseases, provides health professionals with information on the manifestations, pathogenesis, diagnosis, and treatment of scleroderma. Scleroderma represents a group of diseases in which a general process of thickening and induration of the skin results from the excessive deposition of collagen and other matrix proteins. Localized scleroderma refers to asymmetric skin induration and thickening without internal organ involvement. Systemic scleroderma is characterized by fairly symmetric cutaneous induration and thickening, accompanied by visceral organ involvement that may lead to complications. The two major variants of localized scleroderma are morphea and linear scleroderma. Morphea is characterized by circumscribed, indurated, round or ill-defined patches of skin with varying degrees of pigmentary change. The linear variant affects the extremities more commonly than the trunk and is almost always asymmetric. There is no specific therapy for localized scleroderma, although topical corticosteroids, antimalarials, and vitamins D and E have been effective in treating morphea. Most patients require only an emollient for dry skin. Limited systemic scleroderma is characterized by disseminated telangiectasias and sclerodermatous skin changes limited to the hands, forearms, and face. In diffuse systemic scleroderma, Raynaud's phenomenon and systemic rheumatologic, cardiac, neurologic, gastrointestinal, and pulmonary symptoms are common. Treatment of systemic scleroderma is aimed at improving quality of life. Vasoactive therapy includes nicotinic acid, dipyridamole, and calcium channel blockers. Anti-inflammatory therapy consists mainly of oral corticosteroids. Agents used to influence connective tissue metabolism include immunosuppressives and D-penicillamine. Localized scleroderma is typically a self-limited disease that lasts between 3 and 5 years. Systemic scleroderma is chronic, with a slow course of progressive morbidity and disability in 70 to 90 percent of patients. 2 figures, 5 tables, and 15 references. (AA-M).

- **Cutaneous Manifestations of Rheumatic Diseases: Lupus Erythematosus, Dermatomyositis, Scleroderma**

Source: Dermatology Nursing. 10(2): 81-95. April 1998.

Summary: This journal article presents nurses and other health professionals with information, which is part of a continuing education series, on recognizing and managing the cutaneous manifestations of rheumatic diseases. It discusses the classification, diagnosis, clinical features, and management of skin disease seen in patients with lupus erythematosus (LE), dermatomyositis (DM), and scleroderma/systemic sclerosis. The cutaneous manifestations of LE can be divided into those that are histologically specific and those that are not. Each LE-specific skin disease produces a particular type of skin lesion. Patients with LE are photosensitive, so they should protect their skin from sun exposure. In addition, patients with LE may be treated with topical and intralesional corticosteroids, antimalarials, nonimmunosuppressive anti-inflammatory drugs, and immunosuppressives. A cautious approach should be used with regard to surgery. DM is characterized by skin lesions and a histopathologically specific pattern of skeletal muscle inflammation. Patients should use sunscreens, and they may be treated with topical antipruritics, antihistamines, antimalarials, prednisone, and other drugs. Scleroderma, which has two forms, is characterized by thickened, hardened, leather-like skin. The initial manifestation of localized scleroderma is asymmetrical circumscribed indurated plaques on the truck or proximal extremities that are often surrounded by a halo of violaceous skin. Systemic sclerosis, the second form, usually begins with Raynaud's phenomenon. The same moisturization and antipruritic measures described for DM should be used for scleroderma: that is systemic antibiotics, vasodilators, anticoagulants, immunosuppressive drugs, and various investigational approaches. 8 figures, 7 tables, and 21 references.

- **Association of Microsatellite Markers Near the Fibrillin 1 Gene on Human Chromosome 15q With Scleroderma in a Native American Population**

Source: Arthritis and Rheumatism. 41(10): 1729-1737. October 1998.

Summary: This journal article provides health professionals with information on a case control study that investigated the association of microsatellite alleles on human chromosome 15q and 2q with scleroderma in an American Indian population. Microsatellite alleles on these chromosomes, homologous to the murine tight skin 1 (tsk1) and tsk2 loci, respectively, were analyzed for possible disease association in 18 Choctaw patients with systemic sclerosis (SSc) and 77 normal Choctaw controls. Genotyping first-degree relatives of the cases identified potential disease haplotypes, and haplotype frequencies were obtained by expectation maximization and maximum likelihood estimation methods. Simultaneously, the ancestral origins of contemporary Choctaw SSc cases were ascertained using census and historical records. A multilocus 2 cM haplotype identified on human chromosome 15q homologous to the murine tsk1 region, which showed a significantly increased frequency in SSc cases compared with controls. This haplotype contains two intragenic markers from the fibrillin 1 (FBN1) gene. Genealogic studies demonstrate that the SSc cases were distantly related and that their ancestry could be traced back to five founding families in the eighteenth century. The probability that the SSc cases share this haplotype because of familial aggregation effects alone was calculated and found to be very low. There was no evidence of any microsatellite allele disturbances on chromosome 2q in the region homologous to the tsk2 locus of the region containing the interleukin 1 family. The article concludes that a 2 cM haplotype on chromosome 15q that contains FBN1 is associated with scleroderma in Choctaw Indians from Oklahoma. This haplotype may have been inherited from common founders about 10 generations ago and may contribute to the high prevalence of SSC that is now seen. 1 appendix, 1 figure, 3 tables, and 59 references. (AA-M).

- **Classification and Epidemiology of Scleroderma**

Source: Seminars in Cutaneous Medicine and Surgery. 17(1): 22-26. March 1998.

Summary: This journal article provides health professionals with information on the classification and epidemiology of localized and systemic scleroderma. Both forms of scleroderma share many of the same clinical and histological features. The classification scheme for morphea or localized scleroderma divides morphea into plaque, generalized, bullous, linear, and deep. Using this classification system, the incidence rate of localized scleroderma is estimated to be 27 new cases per million population per year. Overall survival is similar to that of the general population. There is a preponderance of female cases for all forms of morphea except for linear scleroderma, which has an even distribution by sex. Systemic scleroderma is divided into limited and diffuse disease depending on the extent of skin involvement. Limited disease is defined as skin involvement confined to areas distal to the elbows and knees, whereas diffuse disease is defined as skin involvement extending above the elbows or above the knees. Recent estimates have placed the incidence rate of systemic sclerosis in the United States at 19 new cases per million adults per year, with an overall prevalence of 240 per million adults. The female-to-male ratio is approximately 5 to 1. The prevalence of scleroderma varies by geographic region and ethnic background and is higher in the United States than in Europe or Japan. Although survival has improved over the past two decades, with 5-year survival over 80 percent, long-term survival is significantly lower than expected, and morbidity is high. 3 tables and 54 references. (AA-M).

- **Clinical Manifestations of Systemic Sclerosis**

  Source: Seminars in Cutaneous Medicine and Surgery. 17(1): 48-54. March 1998.

  Summary: This journal article provides health professionals with information on the clinical manifestations of systemic sclerosis. This chronic multisystem disorder is characterized by inflammation and fibrosis of many organs. Most patients can easily be classified into one of the two main subsets, limited scleroderma and diffuse scleroderma. Patients who have limited cutaneous scleroderma, the old CREST syndrome, generally have Raynaud's phenomenon for a long duration before other symptoms develop. They have skin thickening limited to hands and frequently have problems with digital ulcers and esophageal dysmotility. Although this is generally a milder form than diffuse scleroderma, patients can have life threatening complications from small intestine hypomotility and pulmonary hypertension. Conversely, patients who have diffuse cutaneous scleroderma have a much more acute onset, with many constitutional symptoms, arthritis, carpal tunnel syndrome, and marked swelling of hands and legs. They get widespread skin thickening that progresses from their fingers to their trunk. Internal organ problems, including gastrointestinal and pulmonary fibrosis, are common, but severe life threatening involvement of the heart and kidneys also occurs. Understanding the type of disease that occurs in these two subsets will enable the physician to anticipate problems, aggressively treat those that can be treated, and give patients a better understanding of their disease. 2 tables and 19 references. (AA-M).

- **Effective Intervention in Scleroderma Renal Crisis**

  Source: Journal of Musculoskeletal Medicine. 14(3): 25-28,34-36; March 1997.

  Summary: This journal article for health professionals discusses recent advances in aborting scleroderma renal crisis; however, these advances are possible only with early diagnosis and treatment with angiotensin converting enzyme (ACE) inhibitors. Once irreversible and invariably fatal, scleroderma renal crisis is now considered a treatable complication of systemic sclerosis. Patients with early, rapidly progressive diffuse systemic sclerosis and those with symptomatic pericardial disease and microangiopathic hemolytic anemia are at highest risk. Early recognition and immediate initiation of therapy with captopril or another short-acting ACE inhibitor may be lifesaving. One-year patient survival, once unheard of, has increased to approximately 75 percent. Patients at risk must be educated in self-monitoring of blood pressure and recognition of the early warning signs of renal crisis. If treatment of renal crisis is delayed, long-term dialysis may be required pending the possible return of renal function. 19 references, 2 figures, and 3 tables. (AA-M).

- **Guidelines of Care for Scleroderma and Sclerodermoid Disorders**

Source: Journal of the American Academy of Dermatology. 35(4):609-614; October 1996.

Summary: This journal article for health professionals presents guidelines of care for scleroderma and sclerodermoid disorders. Types of primary cutaneous sclerosis and secondary cutaneous sclerosis are identified. The rationale for the guidelines is presented. Guidelines for obtaining clinical information on systemic sclerosis (SSc) and localized scleroderma are outlined, and tests that may be useful in the diagnosis of scleroderma and localized scleroderma are highlighted. Recommendations concerning the treatment of SSc and localized scleroderma are presented, focusing on topical and systemic therapy, surgery, and evolving therapies. Suggestions for patient education, consultation with other professionals, and aesthetic rehabilitation are also provided for SSc. 22 references.

- **Childhood-onset Scleroderma: Is It Different From Adult-onset Disease?**

Source: Arthritis and Rheumatism. 39(6):1041-1049; June 1996.

Summary: This journal article for health professionals describes a study that explored the differences between childhood-onset scleroderma and adult-onset disease. The clinical and serologic features of 58 patients with childhood-onset scleroderma were examined in the largest cohort of such patients studied to date. These parameters were compared with data obtained from patients with adult-onset disease. Results indicate that childhood-onset scleroderma resembled adult- onset disease with regard to the heterogeneity of clinical expression and subsets of disease, but it also differed from adult-onset disease in a number of clinical and laboratory parameters. The predominant childhood-onset disease presentation was the localized form of the disease, with limited and diffuse systemic sclerosis being less notable. There was a significant association of trauma with childhood-onset scleroderma, which was not noted in adult-onset disease. Furthermore, in contrast to adult disease, patients with childhood-onset disease had normal levels of parameters of vascular activation, T cell activation, and collagen synthesis; a notable lack of antocentromere antibodies; and abnormal coagulation indices. Results, therefore, demonstrate that several features distinguish childhood-onset scleroderma from adult-onset disease. 58 references and 4 tables. (AA-M).

- **Long-Term Outcomes of Scleroderma Renal Crisis**

  Source: Annals of Internal Medicine. 133(8): 600-603. October 17, 2000.

  Contact: Available from American College of Physicians. American Society of Internal Medicine. 190 North Independence Mall West, Philadelphia, PA 19106-1572. Website: www.acponline.org.

  Summary: Although scleroderma renal (kidney) crisis, a complication of systemic sclerosis, can be treated with ACE (angiotensin converting enzyme) inhibitors, its long term outcomes are not known. This article reports on a study undertaken to determine outcomes, natural history, and risk factors in patients with systemic sclerosis and scleroderma renal crisis. The study included 145 patients with scleroderma renal crisis who received ACE inhibitors and 662 patients with scleroderma who did not have renal crisis. Among patients with renal crisis, 61 percent had good outcomes (55 received no dialysis, and 34 received temporary dialysis); only 4 (4 percent) of these patients progressed to chronic renal failure (CRF) and permanent dialysis. More than half of the patients who initially required dialysis could discontinue it 3 to 18 months later. Survival of patients in the good outcome group was similar to that of patients with diffuse scleroderma who did not have renal crisis. Some patients (39 percent) had bad outcomes (permanent dialysis or early death). The authors conclude that renal crisis can be effectively managed when hypertension is aggressively controlled with ACE inhibitors. Patients should continue taking ACE inhibitors even after beginning dialysis in hopes of discontinuing dialysis. 2 figures. 13 references.

Federally-Funded Research on Scleroderma

The U.S. Government supports a variety of research studies relating to scleroderma and associated conditions. These studies are tracked by the

Office of Extramural Research at the National Institutes of Health.[20] CRISP (Computerized Retrieval of Information on Scientific Projects) is a searchable database of federally-funded biomedical research projects conducted at universities, hospitals, and other institutions. Visit the CRISP Web site at **http://commons.cit.nih.gov/crisp3/CRISP.Generate_Ticket**.   You   can perform targeted searches by various criteria including geography, date, as well as topics related to scleroderma and related conditions.

For most of the studies, the agencies reporting into CRISP provide summaries or abstracts. As opposed to clinical trial research using patients, many federally-funded studies use animals or simulated models to explore scleroderma and related conditions. In some cases, therefore, it may be difficult to understand how some basic or fundamental research could eventually translate into medical practice. The following sample is typical of the type of information found when searching the CRISP database for scleroderma:

- **Project Title: CD40L/CD40 Interactions in Scleroderma--Potential Anti CD40L Trial**

  Principal Investigator & Institution: Yellin, Michael J.; Columbia University Health Sciences Ogc New York, Ny 10032

  Timing: Fiscal Year 2000

  Summary: In this grant proposal we plan to study the role of CD154-CD40 interactions in orchestrating inflammation and fibrosis in scleroderma. Additional, we will utilize new technology to study the TCR repertoire and antigen specificity of T cells cloned from dermal lesions of patients with scleroderma. Scleroderma is an autoimmune disease characterized by endothelial cell and fibroblast activation resulting in obliterative vasculopathy and fibrosis. Antigen activated CD4+ T cells play central roles in orchestrating the inflammation and fibrosis characteristic of the disease. The identity of antigens driving the cellular immune response in tissues of patients are not known. Additionally, the T cell effector antigens driving the cellular immune response in tissues of patients are not known. Additionally, the T cell effector molecules regulating inflammation and tissue injury in scleroderma are not precisely known but it is likely that CD154 mediated signals participate in the process. In this regard, CD154 is an activation

---

[20] Healthcare projects are funded by the National Institutes of Health (NIH), Substance Abuse and Mental Health Services (SAMHSA), Health Resources and Services Administration (HRSA), Food and Drug Administration (FDA), Centers for Disease Control and Prevention (CDCP), Agency for Healthcare Research and Quality (AHRQ), and Office of Assistant Secretary of Health (OASH).

induced cell surface molecule predominantly expressed on antigen activated CD4+ T cells. The CD154 counter-receptor is CD40, expressed on a variety of cells, including endothelial cells and fibroblast. CD154-CD40 interactions play key roles in both humoral and cellular immune responses and blocking CD154 mediated signals in vivo inhibits murine models of systemic lupus erythematosis and rheumatoid arthritis. With regard to potential roles in regulating cellular immune responses, we have previously demonstrated that CD40 ligation induces endothelial cell and fibroblast activation. In more recent studies, we have demonstrated that CD154-CD40 interactions induce fibroblasts and endothelial cells to secrete prostaglandins and/or leukocyte chemoattractants. Moreover, CD154 mediated signals appear to regulate leukocyte migration in vivo because anti-CD154 mAB therapy prevents the perivascular accumulation of inflammatory cells in the murine bleomycin induced pulmonary fibrosis model. Evidence for CD154-CD40 interactions playing pathogenic roles in scleroderma is provided by our observation of infiltrating CD154+ lymphocytes in dermal biopsy specimens from patients with scleroderma. Because T cells and T cell effector molecules in particular CD154, are likely key mediators of scleroderma pathogenesis, we plan the following studies: 1) characterize the functional role of CD40 on scleroderma fibroblasts in vitro. In particular, we will determine if CD154-CD40 interactions modulate fibroblast growth, extracellular matrix production or chemokine secretion. 2) Utilize the technology provided in Core Laboratories A and B of this project to clone T cells from dermal lesions and characterize the TCR repertoire and antigen specificity of the cells.. In particular, T cells will be immortalized with herpes virus saimairi (HVS). HVS immortalized cells grow indefinitely in culture and retain there antigen specificity. 3) pilot a study of anti-CD154 mAb in treating early diffuse scleroderma. We plan to study the efficacy of a humanized anti-CD154 mAb, initially developed at Columbia, in modulating the cellular performance and humoral immune responses and clinical outcome in patients.

Website: http://commons.cit.nih.gov/crisp3/CRISP.Generate_Ticket

- **Project Title: Differential Gene Expression in Scleroderma Fibroblasts**

Principal Investigator & Institution: Strehlow, David R.; Research Assistant Professor; Medicine; Boston University 121 Bay State Rd Boston, Ma 02215

Timing: Fiscal Year 2000; Project Start 1-SEP-2000; Project End 0-JUN-2003

Summary: The underlying basis of systemic sclerosis, scleroderma, is unknown. Cultured dermal fibroblasts from scleroderma patients overexpress extracellular matrix components, thus retaining a feature of scleroderma skin in the culture model. We used differential display and hybridization to large arrays of expressed sequence tags to compare gene expression in scleroderma and healthy fibroblasts. Our recently published data show that protease nexin 1, a protein that regulates matrix metabolism, is expressed in scleroderma skin but not in skin from healthy individuals. Because protease nexin 1 is known to inhibit the activation of collagenase, and because we have shown that protease nexin 1 induces collagen transcription, we created transgenic mice containing the human protease nexin 1 cDNA in a cytomegalovirus transcription unit. Part of the current proposal is to examine these mice as a potential model of fibrotic disease. We recently found another gene with more dramatic differential expression. Hybridization to large arrays of expressed sequence tags demonstrated that heat shock protein 90 (hsp90) is overexpressed in scleroderma fibroblasts. Northern analysis showed that hsp90 is highly expressed in scleroderma fibroblasts and not detected in healthy fibroblasts. Overexpression in healthy cells or heat shock itself caused a significant increase in endogenous collagen message. Overexpression of hsp90 also causes a 3.6-fold reduction in collagenase promoter activity (MMP1). Furthermore, a specific inhibitor of hsp90, geldanamycin, obliterates TGFbeta-induced collagen transcription. Hsp90 is known as a molecular chaperone. The chaperone activity of hsp90 is essential to the normal function of the hormone receptor. TGFbeta activates a receptor system, which in turn causes phosphorylation of a cytoplasmic protein called Smad. Phosphorylation of Smad causes its transport to the nucleus where it binds to a specific transcriptional regulatory sequence. Our recent novel finding is that hsp90 is a component of the Smad signaling complex. The second aim of this proposal is therefore to more firmly understand the overexpression of hsp90 in scleroderma skin. The final aim in this proposal is to define the nature of the interactions between Smad, hsp90 and related proteins in the Smad signaling complex and thus to understand how hsp90 functions in regarding TGF-beta signaling.

Website: http://commons.cit.nih.gov/crisp3/CRISP.Generate_Ticket

- **Project Title: Fine Specificity of Scleroderma Autoantibodies**

Principal Investigator & Institution: James, Judith A.; Associate Professor; Oklahoma Medical Research Foundation 825 Ne 13Th St, Ms 31 Oklahoma City, Ok 73104

Timing: Fiscal Year 2001; Project Start 6-SEP-2001; Project End 1-MAY-2006

Summary: (provided by applicant): Systemic sclerosis (scleroderma) is a disfiguring, multi-system disease of unknown etiology, which is characterized by a broad spectrum of disease manifestations with varying organ involvement. Raynaud's phenomenon, the dysregulated vascular contraction of the terminal arteries of the circulatory system, is present in almost every case. Vascular insufficiency in these patients is associated with a vasculopathy causing tissue ischemia, which is directly linked to progressive fibrosis of specific target organs, such as the skin, lung, heart, gastrointestinal tract, and kidney. Although the underlying pathophysiology of this disorder remains an enigma, the presence of anti-nuclear antibodies in scleroderma patients is nearly universal. Targets of these autoantibodies include topoisomerase 1 (Scl-70), nuclear ribonucleoproteins (nRNP), centromere, PM-Scl, and Ku. Anti-topoisomerase-1 (topo-1) autoantibodies are quite specific for scleroderma. and are present in precipitating levels in 20-40% of patients. Anti-topo 1 is associated with diffuse skin thickening, lung involvement, and the development of lung, colon, and brain cancer. Scleroderma patients with anti-nRNP autoantibodies may have a more cutaneous form of the disease and universally suffer from Raynaud's phenomenon. Over the past decade we have extensively characterized the immunochemistry of lupus autoantigens. These previous studies provide the technical background for this proposal. Epitope mapping experiments of the lupus spliceosomal autoantigens have led to a peptide induced model of lupus autoimmunity. These studies have identified a potential etiological trigger and pathogenic mechanisms. We will now apply these well-honed techniques, as well as a similar scientific strategy, to analyze the humoral fine specificity of the anti-nRNP and anti-topoisomerase autoantibodies found in scleroderma. Preliminary data suggest a dramatic difference in the anti-nRNP response of SLE patients and scleroderma patients with nRNP autoantibodies. This project seeks to identify the common humoral epitopes of nRNP and topoisomerase-1 in scleroderma and primary Raynaud's, to describe the development of these humoral autoimmune responses over time (and with therapy), to establish potential etiological triggers of these rheumatic diseases, and to understand the role of these specific autoantibodies in scleroderma, disease pathogenesis.

Website: http://commons.cit.nih.gov/crisp3/CRISP.Generate_Ticket

- **Project Title: Genetic Vs Environment in Scleroderma Outcomes Study**

  Principal Investigator & Institution: Reveille, John D.; University of Texas Hlth Sci Ctr Houston Box 20036 Houston, Tx 77225

Timing: Fiscal Year 2001; Project Start 5-SEP-1997; Project End 1-AUG-2006

Summary: The hypothesis to be tested in this proposal is that systemic sclerosis (SSC) is a more aggressive disease in non-Caucasians who manifest a higher occurrence of critical organ involvement and a worse prognosis, and that reasons for this may include both genetic factor factors as well as sociodemographic or behavioral determinants. To ascertain this we have established a multi-ethic cohort of 175 patients with SSC of relatively recent onset (<five years) deemed the GENISOS cohort (Genetics versus Environment In Scleroderma Outcome Study) which are following at regular intervals. Our specific aims are: 1) To continue followup of the GENISOS cohort of Caucasians, Hispanics and African Americans with SSc of five years of less duration at the University of Texas Health Science Center at Houston, the University of Texas Medical Branch at Galveston and the University of Texas Health Science Center at San Antonio in order to follow their course and outcome at regular intervals for a period of five to seven years and to enroll 80 new cases at the three centers, focusing especially on African American patients. 2) To determine the HLA class II genotypes (HLA-DRB1, DQA1, DQB1 and DPB1 alleles) as well as disease-associated alleles of other candidate genes found to be associated with SSc in ongoing studies in our Division and elsewhere (e.g. fibrillin, SPARC, and others). 3) To determine the sociodemographic parameters (income, education, insurance status) and behavioral features (illness behavior, health care utilization and attitudes, compliance) of these patients. 4) To determine pertinent clinical and laboratory parameters, including disease manifestations (e.g. extent of organ system involvement and co-morbidities), laboratory features (CBC, urinalysis, serum creatinine, serial pulmonary function tests, high resolution CT(HRCT), chest Xray and selected SSc-associated autoantibodies (anti-centromere antibodies (ACA), anti-topoisomerase I (anti-topo I), anti-fibrillin (anti-fib, etc) whose expression has been shown to e associated with specific clinical features of SSc as well as with certain HLA class II alleles. 5) To follow disease progression to outcomes manifested by: a) the development of end-stage pulmonary fibrosis (manifested by a forced vital capacity of 3.0 mg/dl not drug related; c) scleroderma heart disease, defined as either congestive heart failure (defined as a left ventricular ejection fraction of <40%) or malignant arrhythmias requiring therapy; d) functional disability (determined by the SF36 and the mHAQ); e) skin score; f) cumulative disease damage (as measured by the Disease Severity Scale proposed by Medsger et al (1) or death. 6) To examine how gene expression (of fibroblasts from involved and uninvolved skin and from peripheral blood leukocytes) at one point early in disease course predict disease progression (using the outcomes stated above). 7) To examine the relative contributions and interactions of genetic, demographic, socioeconomic, cultural, family history and initial and followup clinical and laboratory features on the course and outcome of early SSc through time dependent statistical analytic approaches including proportional hazard Cox-regression models and longitudinal analysis methods. By elucidating the sociodemographic, behavioral and genetic contributions to morbidity and mortality in SSC, interventions would be possible that could improve the course and outcome of this disease.

Website: http://commons.cit.nih.gov/crisp3/CRISP.Generate_Ticket

- **Project Title: Immune Recognition of Modified Antigen in Scleroderma**

  Principal Investigator & Institution: Hoffman, Robert W.; Professor; Internal Medicine; University of Missouri Columbia 105 Jesse Hall Columbia, Mo 65211

  Timing: Fiscal Year 2001; Project Start 1-SEP-2001; Project End 1-MAY-2004

  Summary: (provided by applicant): Small nuclear ribonucleoproteins (snRNP) are prominent self antigens targeted in scleroderma and other autoimmune conditions. The overall goal of this proposal is to characterize the role of antibodies directed against snRNP in the pathogenesis of scleroderma. In recent work, we have shown that patients who recognize the oxidative modified form of 70k have scleroderma-spectrum clinical characteristics. Furthermore, we have demonstrated that the lupus-associated apoptotic form of 70k is antigenically distinct from intact 70k. We hypothesize that oxidative modified 70k exposes previously cryptic epitopes, driving the development of scleroderma-associated anti-70k immune response. This proposal will seek to test this hypothesis and define the antigenetically distinct epitopes of oxidative 70k recognized by human anti-snRNP antibodies. The four Specific Aims of this proposal are: 1) identify antibodies that specifically bind at high affinity to oxidative 70k but not to native or apoptotic 70k from scleroderma-spectrum disease patient sera; 2) define the structural modification of 70k produced by metal-catalyzed oxidation that are sufficient to induce exposure of oxidative-specific 70k epitopes; 3) map oxidative-specific 70k antibody epitopes; 4) generate monoclonal anti-oxidative 70k antibodies from phage display expression libraries. To accomplish Aim 1, we will examine at least 40 sera known to have anti-70k antibodies from our large well-characterized cohort of patients using oxidative 70k and immunoblotting. Specificity will be determined in blocking studies using molar excess of either intact, apoptotic 70k or oxidative modified 70k pre-incubated prior to immunoblotting. We anticipate that we will be able to define a panel of patients with oxidative-specific antibodies. In Aim 2, we will use expression cloning and site-directed mutagenesis to define the products of 70k produced by metal-catalyzed oxidation. We anticipate that we will be able to define the sites of 70k that preferentially express oxidative-specific epitopes. In Aim 3, we will use truncation and point mutation of the 70k fusion protein, along with synthetic polypeptides and oxidative-specific 70k antibodies, to define the linear B cell epitopes on oxidative-modified 70k. We predict that these experiments will serve to define the B cell epitope on oxidative-modified 70k and anticipate that this will reside in p94-194 region of 70k. Finally, in Aim 4, we will use phage Fab expression libraries to identify antibodies that specifically bind at high affinity to oxidative 70k. We anticipate that these experiments will determine whether heavy and light chain gene usage patterns are similar between libraries generated from different patients. These Fab may then serve as valuable reagents for a series of future experiments derived directly from the work proposed.

Website: http://commons.cit.nih.gov/crisp3/CRISP.Generate_Ticket

- **Project Title: Integrin Alpha1beta1 and Scleroderma**

Principal Investigator & Institution: Gardner, Humphrey A.; Scripps Research Institute 10550 N Torrey Pines Rd San Diego, Ca 92037

Timing: Fiscal Year 2000; Project Start 1-JAN-1998; Project End 1-DEC-2002

Summary: Scleroderma is a devastating connective tissue disease. An increase in dermal collagen synthesis is central to its pathogenesis. This increase has been linked to deficiency of the integrin collagen receptor alpha1 beta1 (a1b1) in scleroderma fibroblasts, and also to an excess of dermal transforming growth factor-beta (TGFb). Studies of normal fibroblasts suggest that integrin a1b1 senses extracellular matrix collagen and mediates feedback inhibition on collagen synthesis. It has also been shown that TGFb causes upregulation of integrin a1b1 in some cell types. The applicants therefore propose that: 1) Increased collagen deposition in scleroderma is due to lack of the normal feedback inhibition of synthesis mediated by integrin a1b1, and 2) that the reduced levels of a1b1 seen in scleroderma fibroblasts may be due to an aberrant response to TGFbeta. Studies are proposed that will enable determination of the role of integrin a1b1 in scleroderma, and which may suggest routes for pharmacologic intervention at a key step in fibrosis. The investigators have generated mice deficient in integrin a1 by gene targeting. These animals develop normally and are fertile. Fibroblasts derived from these animals show increased synthesis of collagen I mRNA compared to wild type. The applicants will examine collagen turnover in these animals by complementary in vitro and in vivo approaches. The applicants will compare collagen synthesis by a1b1-deficient and wild-type fibroblasts in monolayer culture and in 3D gels, and examine the effect on collagen synthesis of addition to these cells of a1 antibody, a1 ligands, and TGFbeta. They will examine collagen synthesis and degradation in the skin of a1b1-deficient and wild-type animals and determine whether the fibrotic effects of TGFb injection are augmented by a1 deficiency. They will isolate alterations in collagen synthesis from alterations in collagen breakdown in vivo by crossing a1-deficient mice with collagenase-resistant mice. They will thus obtain a sensitive assay for the role of a1b1 in regulating collagen synthesis in vivo. These studies will enable them to determine the role of integrin a1b1 in scleroderma and may direct them in the future to dissect the a1 signaling pathway as a target for anti-fibrotic agents.

Website: http://commons.cit.nih.gov/crisp3/CRISP.Generate_Ticket

- **Project Title: Pilot Investigation of the Safety and Efficacy of Thalidomide in Scleroderma**

Principal Investigator & Institution: Oliver, Stephen J.; Rockefeller University 66Th and York Ave New York, Ny 10021

Timing: Fiscal Year 2000

Summary: Scleroderma is a connective tissue disease of unknown etiology characterized by excessive fibrosis of the skin and visceral organs. Scleroderma patients have not responded to traditional immunosuppressive and anti-inflammatory regimens, and the majority of these patients experience progressive disease with marked morbidity and mortality. Chronic graft versus host disease that occurs in bone marrow transplant patients shares many characteristics with scleroderma. In addition, recent reports have suggested that maternal-fetal exchange of cells across placental membranes and persistent microchimerism may contribute to scleroderma pathogenesis. The drug thalidomide, previously known for its teratogenic effects in the early 1960's, has since been found to have anti-inflammatory and immune-modulating effects in a number of immune mediated diseases, including graft-versus-host disease. Furthermore, preliminary studies suggest that the conventional treatment of graft-versus-host disease, cyclosporin A, may be effective in treating scleroderma. Thalidomide use has not been reported in scleroderma patients. This pilot study will obtain preliminary data on the safety and tolerability of thalidomide in scleroderma patients by establishing baseline clinical and serological profiles of patients and then follow those parameters during daily exposure to thalidomide over an initial dose escalation course over 12 weeks, with continued maintenance therapy for up to one year.

Website: http://commons.cit.nih.gov/crisp3/CRISP.Generate_Ticket

- **Project Title: Predicting Pulmonary Hypertension in Scleroderma**

Principal Investigator & Institution: Chang, Betty; Environmental Health Sciences; Johns Hopkins University 3400 N Charles St Baltimore, Md 21218

Timing: Fiscal Year 2001; Project Start 1-SEP-2001

Summary: (provided by applicant): Scleroderma patients with symptomatic pulmonary hypertension (PHTN) have a mean survival of one year; there is limited effective therapy and no way to determine who is at risk. If physicians could predict risk, early intervention could be directed toward those at highest risk. Using a cohort of more tha 950 patients seen at the Johns Hopkins and University of Maryland Scleroderma Center, we propose the following. Specif Aim 1: To differentiate the subpopulations of patients with PHTN using a cross-sectional analysis. We plan to test the hypothesis that the subpopulation of patients with combined pulmonary fibrosis and hypertension have distinctive clinical and demographic features and a worse prognosis than those with isolated PHTN. Specific Aim 2: To ascertain the clinical and demographic features than predict severe PHTN as a complication of scleroderma using a retrospective, longitudinal cohort study of patients who present without PHTN. We hypothesize that PHTN is a vascular abnormality preceded by other vascular symptoms such as severe Raynaud?s leading to amputation. We intend to determine the features associated with severe PHTN. Specific Aim 3: To assess the relationship between lung function measures, patient disease characteristics, and PHTN using a longitudinal cohort of scleroderma patients. The nature of the Diffusion Capacity of Carbon Monoxide (DLCO) relationship with PHTN is unclear. We believe that early changes in DLCO will predict PHTN risk. Specific Aim 4: To determine if anti-fibrillarin antibody is an early marker of severe PHTN by a nested case control study of patients who develop PHTN. We hypothesize that this serum marker can be used to predict who is at high risk for PHTN. With these specific aims, we hope to develop a predictive model for risk assessment for severe PHTN; this is critical to direct early intervention at preventing or delaying hypertension development.

Website: http://commons.cit.nih.gov/crisp3/CRISP.Generate_Ticket

- **Project Title: Studies in Scleroderma and Cystic Fibrosis Osteoporosis**

  Principal Investigator & Institution: Merkel, Peter A.; Assistant Professor; Medicine; Boston University 121 Bay State Rd Boston, Ma 02215

  Timing: Fiscal Year 2001; Project Start 8-JUL-2001; Project End 0-JUN-2006

  Summary: (provided by applicant): To provide support for research projects in the field of rheumatology that will form the basis of a structured mentoring program for young investigators pursuing careers in patient-oriented clinical research. This application has two major specific research aims: 1) Develop new outcome measures for skin assessment in scleroderma for use in clinical trials and 2) Determine the prevalence and progression of osteoporosis in patients with cystic fibrosis (CF). Both projects will have direct relevance to furthering the health of the populations under study. Clinical research in scleroderma, including therapeutic trials, is greatly hampered by a lack of reliable and precise outcome measurements of disease activity. Skin thickening and fibrosis are major causes of morbidity and dysfunction for patients with scleroderma. The great success in extending the life expectancy of patients with CF gained in the last 20 years has resulted in patients now experiencing diseases as adults not formerly encountered in this population. Among these diseases is osteoporosis. Patients with CF appear to be at high risk for osteoporosis due to nutritional, pharmacologic, and genetic factors but the pathophysiology and extent of the problem is not known. Patients with scleroderma will be followed prospectively and evaluated for skin disease activity by skin scoring, durometer readings (thickness), light-based technologies, skin biopsies, self-assessments, and functional status instruments. These data will be analyzed to determine a core set of outcome measures for scleroderma. and validated by an expert panel of national researchers in this disease. An observational cohort of patients with CF will be studied. Baseline and 2-year measurements of bone density, nutritional status, and biochemical markers of bone turnover will performed. A comprehensive program for training new clinical investigators by the principal investigator is proposed. This program includes trainees taking an active and integral role in the research studies described. Additionally, trainees will be enrolled in formal coursework in biostatistics, epidemiology, and clinical research techniques leading to a master degree. A unique seminar and a series of support services at the host institution will further complement the training program.

  Website: http://commons.cit.nih.gov/crisp3/CRISP.Generate_Ticket

- **Project Title: UV-Induced Collagen Reduction--Treating Skin Scleroderma**

Principal Investigator & Institution: Kang, Sewon; Associate Professor; Dermatology; University of Michigan at Ann Arbor Ann Arbor, Mi 48109

Timing: Fiscal Year 2001; Project Start 6-SEP-2001; Project End 0-JUN-2006

Summary: (provided by applicant): Scleroderma is a progressive, potentially life-threatening disease of the connective tissue that can cause hardening of the skin, and damage to lungs, heart, kidney, and gastrointestinal tract, The disease may also affect blood vessels, muscles and joints. Scleroderma typically strikes between ages 25 and 55, and women are four times more likely than men to be stricken. An estimated 300,000 persons in the United States have scleroderma. The exact causes of scleroderma are unknown, however, the hallmark of the disease process is over-production of collagen. Currently, there is no safe and effective therapy for the disease. Acute exposure to relatively low and safe doses of ultraviolet (UV) irradiation has been shown to reduce skin collagen. This reduction occurs through two simultaneous mechanisms; 1) induction of matrix metalloproteinases (MMP) that degrade skin collagen, and 2) inhibit of new procollagen synthesis. UV irradiation is composed of electromagnetic energy with wavelengths between 290-400nm, and the ability of UV to reduce skin collagen is wavelength-dependent. Short wavelengths-dependent between 290-320nm (referred to as UVB) and long wavelengths between 360-400mn (referred to as UVA1) are most effective. In light-colored people, acute exposure to UVB can cause sun turn, and chronic exposure over many years can cause skin cancer. However, the risks of sunburn and cancer from UVA1 are at least one thousand fold less than from UVB exposure. Therefore, UVA1 phototherapy holds great potential for treatment of cutaneous scleroderma in light-colored persons. In dark-colored people, the ability of UV A1 to reduce skin collagen is largely attenuated by skin pigment, likely making this form of phototherapy ineffective. However, for dark-colored people the risk of sunburn and skin cancer from UVB exposure is substantially less than for light-colored people. Therefore, UVB phototherapy for cutaneous scleroderma in dark-colored persons holds great promise. The broad, long-term objectives of this application are to optimize, evaluate, and investigate the molecular basis of UV phototherapy for the treatment of cutaneous scleroderma. The hypothesis that UV irradiation reduces cutaneous fibrosis of scleroderma by inducing MMPS and simultaneously inhibiting procollagen synthesis, and that efficacy of treatment is dependent on patients' skin pigmentation in combination with the UV wavelength used for treatment will be tested. This application contains five specific aims. Specific aims 1-3 focus on optimization of phototherapy conditions based on measurements of collagen reduction. Specific aim 1 will determine the UVA1 dose-, time- and skin color-dependence for induction of a) MMPs, b) tissue inhibitors of MMPs (TIMPS), c) collagen degradation, and d) inhibition of procollagen synthesis in light-pigmented human skin in vivo. Specific aim 2 will determine the broadband (290-320 nm) and narrowband UVB (311-313nm) dose- and time-dependence for reduction of collagen (as described for specific aim 1) in dark-pigmented human skin in vivo. Specific aim 3 will determine the kinetics and magnitude of UVA1-induced tanning, and the impact of this tanning on subsequent UV dose dependence for reduction of collagen (as described for specific aim 1) in lightly-pigmented human skin in vivo. Specific aims 4-5 focus on phototherapy clinical trials for treatment of scleroderma. Specific aim 4 will determine, based on information obtained from Specific Aims 1-3, whether a) an optimized regimen of UVA1 irradiation improves cutaneous scleroderma in light-pigmented patients, and b) an optimized regimen of UVB, improves cutaneous scleroderma in dark-pigmented patients. Specific Aim 5 will determine whether clinical improvement in scleroderma with UV phototherapy correlates with MMP induction, collagen degradation, inhibition of procollagen synthesis, levels of profibrotic (TGF-b, CTGF, IL-4, IL-6) and antifibrotic (TNF-a, IFN-g) cytokines, and infiltrating immune cells.

Website: http://commons.cit.nih.gov/crisp3/CRISP.Generate_Ticket

- **Project Title: Curcumin Treatment of Fibrosis**

Principal Investigator & Institution: Hoffman, Stanley R.; Associate Professor of Medicine and Cell; Medicine; Medical University of South Carolina 171 Ashley Ave Charleston, Sc 29425

Timing: Fiscal Year 2001; Project Start 2-SEP-2001; Project End 0-JUN-2003

Summary: (provided by applicant): Practitioners of alternative medicine recommend curcumin, a component of the spice turmeric, as a treatment for autoimmune diseases. Scleroderma is a debilitating autoimmune disease that affects over 100,000 people in the US, mostly women. The hallmark of scleroderma is dermal fibrosis. When accompanied by visceral organ fibrosis, significant morbidity and mortality results. Despite its widespread occurrence, little is known to suggest effective treatment. As part of our long-term objective of understanding the aberrant regulation of extracellular matrix protein accumulation in scleroderma, we treated primary fibroblast cultures from the lungs of scleroderma patients with curcumin. We found that this treatment inhibits collagen accumulation and promotes cell death in these cultures while having no effect on normal lung fibroblasts. Interestingly, these effects of curcumin on scleroderma fibroblasts are enhanced in the presence of vitamin C. If curcumin were to have the same effect on scleroderma fibroblasts in vivo as it has in culture, then curcumin would be likely to be an effective treatment for scleroderma. While curcumin is not yet used in standard medical practice, in Chinese and Indian folk medicine turmeric is used to treat a broad range of ailments. Published articles show curcumin to have a range of potent biological activities including anticancer, anti-inflammatory, and antimicrobial. The use of curcumin in folk medicine, published studies on curcumin, and our results combine to indicate that curcumin is non-toxic and is a treatment already used in alternative medicine that is likely to have demonstrably positive effects on patients with scleroderma and other fibrotic diseases. In order to test the hypothesis that curcumin may be a beneficial treatment for scleroderma in particular and fibrotic diseases in general, we will: 1) Use cultured fibroblasts to determine the molecular and cellular mechanisms involved in the specific effects of curcumin on cells from scleroderma patients and 2) We will perform translational research using an animal model for scleroderma and lung fibrosis to determine whether curcumin is indeed effective in treating lung fibrosis in vivo. These experiments will demonstrate the efficacy and the scientific basis for that efficacy of a disease treatment already recommended by practitioners of alternative medicine.

Website: http://commons.cit.nih.gov/crisp3/CRISP.Generate_Ticket

- **Project Title: Cytokine Modulation of Collagen Gene Expression: Signal**

Principal Investigator & Institution: Ghosh, Asish; Medicine; University of Illinois at Chicago at Chicago Chicago, Il 60612

Timing: Fiscal Year 2000; Project Start 5-SEP-1999; Project End 1-AUG-2002

Summary: Un controlled accumulation of Type I collagen, the hallmark of scleroderma, results in fibrosis of skin and other affected organs. This process is attributed to constitutive activation of collagen gene transcription in scleroderma fibroblasts, Transforming growth factor-beta (TGF-beta), a potent stimulus for collagen synthesis, is strongly implicated in pathological fibrogenesis , whereas interferon gamma (IFN-gamma) antagonize the effects of TGF-beta and as important for prevention of scarring. Recently, SMAD and STAT1 have been identified as intracellular signal transducers of TGF-beta and IFN-gamma, respectively. However, the pathways for modulating collagen gene transcription in response to these cytokines, and the transcriptional mechanisms involved, remain poorly understood. Our laboratory has established the role of SMAD3 in TGF-beta stimulation of collagen gene regulation of Type I collagen gene transcription, and to delineate alterations that result in its constitutive up-regulation in scleroderma. To this end, building on recent insights from our laboratory relating to TGF-beta and IFN-gamma signaling in fibroblasts and the role of p300/CBP in these pathways, I propose to examine the hypothesis that these co-activators are involved in stimulation as well as inhibition of collagen transcription, and integrate antagonistic signaling to the Typ1 collagen gene promoters. The hypothesis will be tested in the following three Specific Aims: 1) to elucidate the involvement of p300/CBP in activation of Type I collagen transcription by TGF-beta in normal fibroblasts; 2) to dissect the molecular mechanisms underlying antagonistic regulation of collagen gene transcription in these cells by TGF-beta and IFN-gamma; and 3) to examine SMAD-p300/CBP co-activator interactions in scleroderma fibroblasts with constitutive up-regulation of collagen gene transcription. The pilot studies described in this application are based on recent breakthroughs in understanding TGF-beta signaling and the role of co-activators in transcriptional regulation. By enhancing our knowledge of how transcription of collagen genes is regulated in fibroblasts, these studies could ultimately lead to the design of novel therapeutic strategies to selectively modulate this process in Scleroderma.

Website: http://commons.cit.nih.gov/crisp3/CRISP.Generate_Ticket

- **Project Title: Inhibition of Monocyte Tgfb1-Induced Skin Fibrosis**

  Principal Investigator & Institution: Gilliam, Anita C.; Associate Professor; Dermatology; Case Western Reserve University 10900 Euclid Ave Cleveland, Oh 44106

  Timing: Fiscal Year 2000; Project Start 4-JUL-2000; Project End 0-JUN-2003

Summary: The candidate, Anita C. Gilliam, is a junior faculty member on tenure track in Dermatology at Case Western Reserve University (CWRU), where she is developing a research career in molecular mechanisms of autoimmune disease. The proposed work draws on her experience in molecular biology and cutaneous immunobiology, and requests support for a mentored Clinical Scientist Development Award to acquire new expertise in monocyte biology under the mentorship of Dr. Kevin D. Cooper (Dermatology). The research environment, resources, and opportunities for career development at CWRU are superb, with CWRU School of Medicine recently listed as one of the top 10 research institutions in the country, and the Department of Dermatology as the top US program in NIH funding. The candidate's immediate goals are to develop the animal model in the proposed work into a vehicle useful for testing of interventions in scleroderma; long term goals are to develop the science of cutaneous monocyte biology and gene transfer in autoimmune disease as an independently funded investigator in an outstanding research environment. The proposal involves the study of systemic sclerosis/scleroderma, a chronic autoimmune disease of unknown etiology characterized by altered humoral and cell-mediated immunity, and excessive deposition of collagen in viscerae and skin, which is thought to be driven by activated monocytes making TGFbeta. We have characterized a very promising murine model for scleroderma that recapitulates many important features of scleroderma. Hypothesis: Monocytes are critical effector cells in Scl GVHD. TGF -beta1 is a major fibrogenic cytokine driving skin fibrosis in mice with Scl GVHD; TGF-beta2 and TGF-beta3 play minor if any roles in this cutaneous fibrosis. Skin fibrosis can be inhibited by: 1) antibodies to TGF-beta, 2), and latency associated peptide (LAP), a naturally occurring antagonist for TGF-beta. Specific Aim 1: To investigate the mechanism and sequence of early critical events leading to skin fibrosis in animals with Scl GVHD to better understand the pathophysiology of fibrosing disease and to devise novel focused interventions. Establishing the critical parameters of monocyte influx into skin, production of fibrogenic TGFbeta, and upregulation of proalpha(I) collagen mRNA synthesis provides a foundation for in vivo focused interventions. Specific Aim II: To further characterize in vivo interventions that inhibit TGFbeta1 in Scl GVHD. We have shown in preliminary experiments that TGF-beta LAP and antibodies to TGF-beta inhibit skin fibrosis in animals with Scl GVHD. Further characterization of these observations have high relevance to our understanding of basic monocyte biology, to the TGFbeta-driven fibrosing process in the animal model and in the autoimmune disease scleroderma, and potentially to the treatment of scleroderma and human graft versus host disease.

Website: http://commons.cit.nih.gov/crisp3/CRISP.Generate_Ticket

- **Project Title: Regulation of Collagen Gene Expression by TGF Beta**

Principal Investigator & Institution: Varga, John M.; Professor of Medicine; Medicine; University of Illinois at Chicago at Chicago Chicago, Il 60612

Timing: Fiscal Year 2000; Project Start 1-DEC-1993; Project End 0-NOV-2003

Summary: The uncontrolled tissue accumulation of Type I collagen characteristic of scleroderma is attributed to increased transcription of the collagen genes in scleroderma fibroblasts. TGF-Beta, a potent inducer of collagen synthesis, is strongly implicated in the development of pathological fibrosis in scleroderma. Other cytokines such as interferon-gamma antagonize the effects of TGF-Beta, and are likely to be important for prevention of scarring. Little is known about the intracellular signaling pathways involved in the physiologic regulation of collagen synthesis by cytokines, and the cis-acting elements of the collagen genes that are targets for these pathways. This information is of crucial importance for gaining a better understanding of the pathogenesis of fibrosis. We have shown that TGF-Beta stimulates transcription of the alpha1 (I) collagen gene (COL1A1) in fibroblasts. During the previous period of funding, we have identified cis-acting elements and their cognate transcription factors that play roles in regulating basal COL1A1 transcription. Our long-term goal is to understand the cellular mechanisms for modulation of collagen transcription in response to stimulatory and inhibitory extracellular signals, and to delineate alterations in the intracellular signaling pathways that result in constitutive up-regulation of the expression of collagen genes in scleroderma. In Specific Aim 1, we will ask which regions of the human COL1A1 promoter (and first intron) are responsive to TGF-Beta in fibroblasts, and what trans-acting proteins bind to these elements? We will confirm the functional role of TGF-Beta response elements in vivo by gene transfer in mice. In Specific Aim 2, we will examine the role of a novel family of intracellular signaling proteins in activation of collagen transcription by TGF-Beta in vitro. By gain- of-function and loss-of-function experiments, we will ask which Smad proteins are involved, and whether the Smads function as DNA-binding transcription factors in fibroblasts. We will ask if the Smads are molecular targets for antagonistic regulation by cytokines with opposing effects on collagen transcription. In Specific Aim 3, we will ask whether aberrant or deregulated Smad signaling underlies the constitutive up-regulation of collagen transcription in scleroderma fibroblasts. These studies should better define the signaling mechanisms that are important in regulating collagen transcription in normal and fibrotic fibroblasts. The results will facilitate the design of interventions to selectively inhibit this process.

Website: http://commons.cit.nih.gov/crisp3/CRISP.Generate_Ticket

- **Project Title: Relaxin Therapy--Systemic Sclerosis W/ Diffuse Scleroder**

Principal Investigator & Institution: Korn, Joseph H.; Professor; Boston University 121 Bay State Rd Boston, Ma 02215

Timing: Fiscal Year 2000; Project Start 1-DEC-1978; Project End 0-NOV-2001

Summary: The prevalence of systemic sclerosis in the U.S. is estimated to be approximately 68,000, based on a recent epidemiology study published in 1997 which reports a prevalence of 240 cases per million. Systemic sclerosis is three to four times more common in women than in men. Based on the prevalence, systemic sclerosis is an orphan disease and Connetics Corporation has obtained an orphan drug designated for recombinant human relaxin. A non-controlled study conducted in the 1950's using purified porcine relaxin for the treatment of 23 subjects with scleroderma reported some efficacy, particularly in raged to healing of digital ulcers and Raynaud's phenomenon. The ability of ralxin to be evaluated critically for its beneficial effects in this disease was limited by uncertainties concerning the purity of the relaxin preparation sold at this time. The clinical features of scleroderma reflect variable contributions of the pathologic processes of vascular injury, tissue inflammation, secondary fibrosis and ultimately tissue atrophy. Accordingly, this study (RLXN.C.005) employs a variety of assessment techniques and measures which are relevant to judging the clinical status of individuals with systemic sclerosis but which are also reflective of diverse pathologic processes operative in this disorder. These techniques and measures are basis of the experimental design in this trial. The well-defined biologic properties of relaxin would suggest the potential for primary effects on measures of the tissue fibrosis and vascular status and secondarily on tissue atrophy. The study design will be a multicenter, randomized, double-blind, placebo controlled trial. A minimum of 180 and a maximum of 200 subjects diagnosed with systemic sclerosis with diffuse scleroderma will be randomized to six months of continuous subcutaneous infusion treatment to one of three parallel treatment groups in a 2:2:1 ratio, with a minimum of 72 subjects in each in the 25 microgram/kg/day and placebo groups, and 36 subjects in the 10 micrograms/kg/day group. The Boston University School of Medicine / Boston Medical Center is to recruit 20-30 subjects for this study.

Website: http://commons.cit.nih.gov/crisp3/CRISP.Generate_Ticket

E-Journals: PubMed Central[21]

PubMed Central (PMC) is a digital archive of life sciences journal literature developed and managed by the National Center for Biotechnology

---

[21] Adapted from the National Library of Medicine:
http://www.pubmedcentral.nih.gov/about/intro.html.

Information (NCBI) at the U.S. National Library of Medicine (NLM).[22] Access to this growing archive of e-journals is free and unrestricted.[23] To search, go to **http://www.pubmedcentral.nih.gov/index.html#search**, and type "scleroderma" (or synonyms) into the search box. This search gives you access to full-text articles. The following is a sample of items found for scleroderma in the PubMed Central database:

- **Autoantibodies from a Patient with Scleroderma CREST Recognized Kinetochores of the Higher Plant Haemanthus** by J Mole-Bajer, AS Bajer, RP Zinkowski, RD Balczon, and BR Brinkley; 1990 May 1 http://www.pubmedcentral.nih.gov/articlerender.fcgi?rendertype=abstract&artid=53949

- **Bilateral linear scleroderma "en coup de sabre" associated with facial atrophy and neurological complications** by Thilo Gambichler, Alexander Kreuter, Klaus Hoffmann, Falk G. Bechara, Peter Altmeyer, and Thomas Jansen; 2001 http://www.pubmedcentral.nih.gov/articlerender.fcgi?artid=61032

- **Characterization of two scleroderma autoimmune antigens that copurify with human ribonuclease P** by Paul S. Eder, Ramesh Kekuda, Viktor Stolc, and Sidney Altman; 1997 February 18 http://www.pubmedcentral.nih.gov/articlerender.fcgi?artid=19751

- **Isolation and Characterization of cDNA Encoding the 80-kDa Subunit Protein of the Human Autoantigen Ku (p70/p80) Recognized by Autoantibodies from Patients with Scleroderma-Polymyositis Overlap Syndrome** by T Mimori, Y Ohosone, N Hama, A Suwa, M Akizuki, M Homma, AJ Griffith, and JA Hardin; 1990 March 1 http://www.pubmedcentral.nih.gov/articlerender.fcgi?rendertype=abstract&artid=53566

- **Rare Scleroderma Autoantibodies to the U11 Small Nuclear Ribonucleoprotein and to the Trimethylguanosine Cap of U Small Nuclear RNAs** by AC Gilliam and JA Steitz; 1993 July 15 http://www.pubmedcentral.nih.gov/articlerender.fcgi?rendertype=abstract&artid=47016

- **The inhibitory effects of camptothecin, a topoisomerase I inhibitor, on collagen synthesis in fibroblasts from patients with systemic sclerosis**

---

[22] With PubMed Central, NCBI is taking the lead in preservation and maintenance of open access to electronic literature, just as NLM has done for decades with printed biomedical literature. PubMed Central aims to become a world-class library of the digital age.

[23] The value of PubMed Central, in addition to its role as an archive, lies the availability of data from diverse sources stored in a common format in a single repository. Many journals already have online publishing operations, and there is a growing tendency to publish material online only, to the exclusion of print.

by Joanna Czuwara-Ladykowska, Barbara Makiela, Edwin A. Smith, Maria Trojanowska, and Lidia Rudnicka; 2001
http://www.pubmedcentral.nih.gov/articlerender.fcgi?artid=64844

- **Von Willebrand factor propeptide as a marker of disease activity in systemic sclerosis (scleroderma)** by Agneta Scheja, Anita Akesson, Pierre Geborek, Marie Wildt, Claes B. Wollheim, Frank A. Wollheim, and Ulrich M. Vischer; 2001
http://www.pubmedcentral.nih.gov/articlerender.fcgi?artid=30710

The National Library of Medicine: PubMed

One of the quickest and most comprehensive ways to find academic studies in both English and other languages is to use PubMed, maintained by the National Library of Medicine. The advantage of PubMed over previously mentioned sources is that it covers a greater number of domestic and foreign references. It is also free to the public.[24] If the publisher has a Web site that offers full text of its journals, PubMed will provide links to that site, as well as to sites offering other related data. User registration, a subscription fee, or some other type of fee may be required to access the full text of articles in some journals.

To generate your own bibliography of studies dealing with scleroderma, simply go to the PubMed Web site at **www.ncbi.nlm.nih.gov/pubmed**. Type "scleroderma" (or synonyms) into the search box, and click "Go." The following is the type of output you can expect from PubMed for "scleroderma" (hyperlinks lead to article summaries):

- **An objective evaluation of the treatment of systemic scleroderma with disodium EDTA, pyridoxine and reserpine.**
Author(s): Fuleihan FJ, Kurban AK, Abboud RT, Beidas-Jubran N, Farah FS.
Source: The British Journal of Dermatology. 1968 March; 80(3): 184-9. No Abstract Available.
http://www.ncbi.nlm.nih.gov:80/entrez/query.fcgi?cmd=Retrieve&db=PubMed&list_uids=4967134&dopt=Abstract

---

[24] PubMed was developed by the National Center for Biotechnology Information (NCBI) at the National Library of Medicine (NLM) at the National Institutes of Health (NIH). The PubMed database was developed in conjunction with publishers of biomedical literature as a search tool for accessing literature citations and linking to full-text journal articles at Web sites of participating publishers. Publishers that participate in PubMed supply NLM with their citations electronically prior to or at the time of publication.

- **Effect of ethylenediaminetetraacetic acid (EDTA) and tetrahydroxyquinone on sclerodermatous skin. Histologic and chemical studies.**
  Author(s): Keech MK, McCann DS, Boyle AJ, Pinkus H.
  Source: The Journal of Investigative Dermatology. 1966 September; 47(3): 235-46. No Abstract Available.
  http://www.ncbi.nlm.nih.gov:80/entrez/query.fcgi?cmd=Retrieve&db=PubMed&list_uids=4958819&dopt=Abstract

Vocabulary Builder

Aberrant: Wandering or deviating from the usual or normal course. [EU]

Alleles: Mutually exclusive forms of the same gene, occupying the same locus on homologous chromosomes, and governing the same biochemical and developmental process. [NIH]

Anemia: A reduction in the number of circulating erythrocytes or in the quantity of hemoglobin. [NIH]

Anorectal: Pertaining to the anus and rectum or to the junction region between the two. [EU]

Anticoagulants: Agents that prevent blood clotting. Naturally occurring agents in the blood are included only when they are used as drugs. [NIH]

Antigen: Any substance which is capable, under appropriate conditions, of inducing a specific immune response and of reacting with the products of that response, that is, with specific antibody or specifically sensitized T-lymphocytes, or both. Antigens may be soluble substances, such as toxins and foreign proteins, or particulate, such as bacteria and tissue cells; however, only the portion of the protein or polysaccharide molecule known as the antigenic determinant (q.v.) combines with antibody or a specific receptor on a lymphocyte. Abbreviated Ag. [EU]

Antihistamine: A drug that counteracts the action of histamine. The antihistamines are of two types. The conventional ones, as those used in allergies, block the H1 histamine receptors, whereas the others block the H2 receptors. Called also antihistaminic. [EU]

Antimicrobial: Killing microorganisms, or suppressing their multiplication or growth. [EU]

Antipruritic: Relieving or preventing itching. [EU]

Arginine: An essential amino acid that is physiologically active in the L-form. [NIH]

Arteries: The vessels carrying blood away from the heart. [NIH]

Assay: Determination of the amount of a particular constituent of a mixture, or of the biological or pharmacological potency of a drug. [EU]

Atrophy: A wasting away; a diminution in the size of a cell, tissue, organ, or part. [EU]

Autoantigens: Endogenous tissue constituents that have the ability to interact with autoantibodies and cause an immune response. [NIH]

Benign: Not malignant; not recurrent; favourable for recovery. [EU]

Biochemical: Relating to biochemistry; characterized by, produced by, or involving chemical reactions in living organisms. [EU]

Bleomycin: A complex of related glycopeptide antibiotics from Streptomyces verticillus consisting of bleomycin A2 and B2. It inhibits DNA metabolism and is used as an antineoplastic, especially for solid tumors. [NIH]

Bullous: Pertaining to or characterized by bullae. [EU]

Camptothecin: An alkaloid isolated from the stem wood of the Chinese tree, Camptotheca acuminata. This compound selectively inhibits the nuclear enzyme DNA topoisomerase. Several semisynthetic analogs of camptothecin have demonstrated antitumor activity. [NIH]

Cardiac: Pertaining to the heart. [EU]

Coagulation: 1. the process of clot formation. 2. in colloid chemistry, the solidification of a sol into a gelatinous mass; an alteration of a disperse phase or of a dissolved solid which causes the separation of the system into a liquid phase and an insoluble mass called the clot or curd. Coagulation is usually irreversible. 3. in surgery, the disruption of tissue by physical means to form an amorphous residuum, as in electrocoagulation and photocoagulation. [EU]

Constitutional: 1. affecting the whole constitution of the body; not local. 2. pertaining to the constitution. [EU]

Curcumin: A dye obtained from tumeric, the powdered root of Curcuma longa Linn. It is used in the preparation of curcuma paper and the detection of boron. Curcumin appears to possess a spectrum of pharmacological properties, due primarily to its inhibitory effects on metabolic enzymes. [NIH]

Cytokines: Non-antibody proteins secreted by inflammatory leukocytes and some non-leukocytic cells, that act as intercellular mediators. They differ from classical hormones in that they are produced by a number of tissue or cell types rather than by specialized glands. They generally act locally in a paracrine or autocrine rather than endocrine manner. [NIH]

Cytomegalovirus: A genus of the family herpesviridae, subfamily betaherpesvirinae, infecting the salivary glands, liver, spleen, lungs, eyes, and other organs, in which they produce characteristically enlarged cells with intranuclear inclusions. Infection with Cytomegalovirus is also seen as an opportunistic infection in AIDS. [NIH]

Dermis: A layer of vascular connective tissue underneath the epidermis. The surface of the dermis contains sensitive papillae. Embedded in or beneath the dermis are sweat glands, hair follicles, and sebaceous glands. [NIH]

Diffusion: The process of becoming diffused, or widely spread; the spontaneous movement of molecules or other particles in solution, owing to their random thermal motion, to reach a uniform concentration throughout the solvent, a process requiring no addition of energy to the system. [EU]

Distal: Remote; farther from any point of reference; opposed to proximal. In dentistry, used to designate a position on the dental arch farther from the median line of the jaw. [EU]

Dysphagia: Difficulty in swallowing. [EU]

Emollient: Softening or soothing; called also malactic. [EU]

Endogenous: Developing or originating within the organisms or arising from causes within the organism. [EU]

Epitopes: Sites on an antigen that interact with specific antibodies. [NIH]

Extracellular: Outside a cell or cells. [EU]

Extracorporeal: Situated or occurring outside the body. [EU]

Gels: Colloids with a solid continuous phase and liquid as the dispersed phase; gels may be unstable when, due to temperature or other cause, the solid phase liquifies; the resulting colloid is called a sol. [NIH]

Genotype: The genetic constitution of the individual; the characterization of the genes. [NIH]

Griseofulvin: An antifungal antibiotic. Griseofulvin may be given by mouth in the treatment of tinea infections. [NIH]

Haplotypes: The genetic constitution of individuals with respect to one member of a pair of allelic genes, or sets of genes that are closely linked and tend to be inherited together such as those of the major histocompatibility complex. [NIH]

Herpes: Any inflammatory skin disease caused by a herpesvirus and characterized by the formation of clusters of small vesicles. When used alone, the term may refer to herpes simplex or to herpes zoster. [EU]

Humoral: Of, relating to, proceeding from, or involving a bodily humour - now often used of endocrine factors as opposed to neural or somatic. [EU]

Hybridization: The genetic process of crossbreeding to produce a hybrid. Hybrid nucleic acids can be formed by nucleic acid hybridization of DNA and RNA molecules. Protein hybridization allows for hybrid proteins to be formed from polypeptide chains. [NIH]

Hyperbaric: Characterized by greater than normal pressure or weight; applied to gases under greater than atmospheric pressure, as hyperbaric oxygen, or to a solution of greater specific gravity than another taken as a standard of reference. [EU]

Immunochemistry: Field of chemistry that pertains to immunological phenomena and the study of chemical reactions related to antigen stimulation of tissues. It includes physicochemical interactions between antigens and antibodies. [NIH]

Induction: The act or process of inducing or causing to occur, especially the production of a specific morphogenetic effect in the developing embryo through the influence of evocators or organizers, or the production of anaesthesia or unconsciousness by use of appropriate agents. [EU]

Induration: 1. the quality of being hard; the process of hardening. 2. an abnormally hard spot or place. [EU]

Infiltration: The diffusion or accumulation in a tissue or cells of substances not normal to it or in amounts of the normal. Also, the material so accumulated. [EU]

Ischemia: Deficiency of blood in a part, due to functional constriction or actual obstruction of a blood vessel. [EU]

Kinetic: Pertaining to or producing motion. [EU]

Kinetochores: Large multiprotein complexes that bind the centromeres of the chromosomes to the microtubules of the mitotic spindle during metaphase in the cell cycle. [NIH]

Larynx: An irregularly shaped, musculocartilaginous tubular structure, lined with mucous membrane, located at the top of the trachea and below the root of the tongue and the hyoid bone. It is the essential sphincter guarding the entrance into the trachea and functioning secondarily as the organ of voice. [NIH]

Ligation: Application of a ligature to tie a vessel or strangulate a part. [NIH]

Malignant: Tending to become progressively worse and to result in death. Having the properties of anaplasia, invasion, and metastasis; said of tumours. [EU]

Mediator: An object or substance by which something is mediated, such as (1) a structure of the nervous system that transmits impulses eliciting a specific response; (2) a chemical substance (transmitter substance) that induces activity in an excitable tissue, such as nerve or muscle; or (3) a substance released from cells as the result of the interaction of antigen with antibody or by the action of antigen with a sensitized lymphocyte. [EU]

Membrane: A thin layer of tissue which covers a surface, lines a cavity or divides a space or organ. [EU]

Microgram: A unit of mass (weight) of the metric system, being one-millionth of a gram (10-6 gm.) or one one-thousandth of a milligram (10-3 mg.). [EU]

Monocytes: Large, phagocytic mononuclear leukocytes produced in the vertebrate bone marrow and released into the blood; contain a large, oval or somewhat indented nucleus surrounded by voluminous cytoplasm and numerous organelles. [NIH]

Mutagenesis: Process of generating genetic mutations. It may occur spontaneously or be induced by mutagens. [NIH]

Neurologic: Pertaining to neurology or to the nervous system. [EU]

Osteoporosis: Reduction in the amount of bone mass, leading to fractures after minimal trauma. [EU]

Oxidation: The act of oxidizing or state of being oxidized. Chemically it consists in the increase of positive charges on an atom or the loss of negative charges. Most biological oxidations are accomplished by the removal of a pair of hydrogen atoms (dehydrogenation) from a molecule. Such oxidations must be accompanied by reduction of an acceptor molecule. Univalent o. indicates loss of one electron; divalent o., the loss of two electrons. [EU]

Penicillamine: 3-Mercapto-D-valine. The most characteristic degradation product of the penicillin antibiotics. It is used as an antirheumatic and as a chelating agent in Wilson's disease. [NIH]

Perivascular: Situated around a vessel. [EU]

Pharmacologic: Pertaining to pharmacology or to the properties and reactions of drugs. [EU]

Phenytoin: An anticonvulsant that is used in a wide variety of seizures. It is also an anti-arrhythmic and a muscle relaxant. The mechanism of therapeutic action is not clear, although several cellular actions have been described including effects on ion channels, active transport, and general membrane stabilization. The mechanism of its muscle relaxant effect appears to involve a reduction in the sensitivity of muscle spindles to stretch. Phenytoin has been proposed for several other therapeutic uses, but its use has been limited by its many adverse effects and interactions with other drugs. [NIH]

Phosphorylation: The introduction of a phosphoryl group into a compound through the formation of an ester bond between the compound and a phosphorus moiety. [NIH]

Photochemotherapy: Therapy using oral or topical photosensitizing agents with subsequent exposure to light. [NIH]

Phototherapy: Treatment of disease by exposure to light, especially by variously concentrated light rays or specific wavelengths. [NIH]

Pigmentation: 1. the deposition of colouring matter; the coloration or discoloration of a part by pigment. 2. coloration, especially abnormally increased coloration, by melanin. [EU]

Polypeptide: A peptide which on hydrolysis yields more than two amino acids; called tripeptides, tetrapeptides, etc. according to the number of amino acids contained. [EU]

Prednisone: A synthetic anti-inflammatory glucocorticoid derived from cortisone. It is biologically inert and converted to prednisolone in the liver. [NIH]

Prevalence: The total number of cases of a given disease in a specified population at a designated time. It is differentiated from incidence, which refers to the number of new cases in the population at a given time. [NIH]

Procollagen: A biosynthetic precursor of collagen containing additional amino acid sequences at the amino-terminal ends of the three polypeptide chains. Protocollagen, a precursor of procollagen consists of procollagen peptide chains in which proline and lysine have not yet been hydroxylated. [NIH]

Proportional: Being in proportion : corresponding in size, degree, or intensity, having the same or a constant ratio; of, relating to, or used in determining proportions. [EU]

Prostaglandins: A group of compounds derived from unsaturated 20-carbon fatty acids, primarily arachidonic acid, via the cyclooxygenase pathway. They are extremely potent mediators of a diverse group of physiological processes. [NIH]

Protease: Proteinase (= any enzyme that catalyses the splitting of interior peptide bonds in a protein). [EU]

Proximal: Nearest; closer to any point of reference; opposed to distal. [EU]

Reagent: A substance employed to produce a chemical reaction so as to detect, measure, produce, etc., other substances. [EU]

Receptor: 1. a molecular structure within a cell or on the surface characterized by (1) selective binding of a specific substance and (2) a specific physiologic effect that accompanies the binding, e.g., cell-surface receptors for peptide hormones, neurotransmitters, antigens, complement fragments, and immunoglobulins and cytoplasmic receptors for steroid hormones. 2. a sensory nerve terminal that responds to stimuli of various kinds. [EU]

Reflective: Capable of throwing back light, images, sound waves : reflecting. [EU]

Reflux: A backward or return flow. [EU]

Reserpine: An alkaloid found in the roots of Rauwolfia serpentina and R. vomitoria. Reserpine inhibits the uptake of norepinephrine into storage vesicles resulting in depletion of catecholamines and serotonin from central and peripheral axon terminals. It has been used as an antihypertensive and an antipsychotic as well as a research tool, but its adverse effects limit its clinical use. [NIH]

Retinoids: Derivatives of vitamin A. Used clinically in the treatment of severe cystic acne, psoriasis, and other disorders of keratinization. Their possible use in the prophylaxis and treatment of cancer is being actively explored. [NIH]

Secretion: 1. the process of elaborating a specific product as a result of the activity of a gland; this activity may range from separating a specific substance of the blood to the elaboration of a new chemical substance. 2. any substance produced by secretion. [EU]

Serum: The clear portion of any body fluid; the clear fluid moistening serous membranes. 2. blood serum; the clear liquid that separates from blood on clotting. 3. immune serum; blood serum from an immunized animal used for passive immunization; an antiserum; antitoxin, or antivenin. [EU]

Spectrum: A charted band of wavelengths of electromagnetic vibrations obtained by refraction and diffraction. By extension, a measurable range of activity, such as the range of bacteria affected by an antibiotic (antibacterial s.) or the complete range of manifestations of a disease. [EU]

Stasis: A word termination indicating the maintenance of (or maintaining) a constant level; preventing increase or multiplication. [EU]

Sunburn: An injury to the skin causing erythema, tenderness, and sometimes blistering and resulting from excessive exposure to the sun. The reaction is produced by the ultraviolet radiation in sunlight. [NIH]

Teratogenic: Tending to produce anomalies of formation, or teratism (= anomaly of formation or development : condition of a monster). [EU]

Thalidomide: A pharmaceutical agent originally introduced as a non-barbiturate hypnotic, but withdrawn from the market because of its known tetratogenic effects. It has been reintroduced and used for a number of immunological and inflammatory disorders. Thalidomide displays immunosuppresive and anti-angiogenic activity. It inhibits release of tumor necrosis factor alpha from monocytes, and modulates other cytokine action. [NIH]

Thermal: Pertaining to or characterized by heat. [EU]

Thermography: Measurement of the regional temperature of the body or an organ by infrared sensing devices, based on self-emanating infrared radiation. [NIH]

Topical: Pertaining to a particular surface area, as a topical anti-infective applied to a certain area of the skin and affecting only the area to which it is applied. [EU]

Transcutaneous: Transdermal. [EU]

Urinalysis: Examination of urine by chemical, physical, or microscopic means. Routine urinalysis usually includes performing chemical screening tests, determining specific gravity, observing any unusual color or odor, screening for bacteriuria, and examining the sediment microscopically. [NIH]

Vasoactive: Exerting an effect upon the calibre of blood vessels. [EU]

Ventricular: Pertaining to a ventricle. [EU]

CHAPTER 5. PATENTS ON SCLERODERMA

Overview

You can learn about innovations relating to scleroderma by reading recent patents and patent applications. Patents can be physical innovations (e.g. chemicals, pharmaceuticals, medical equipment) or processes (e.g. treatments or diagnostic procedures). The United States Patent and Trademark Office defines a patent as a grant of a property right to the inventor, issued by the Patent and Trademark Office.[25] Patents, therefore, are intellectual property. For the United States, the term of a new patent is 20 years from the date when the patent application was filed. If the inventor wishes to receive economic benefits, it is likely that the invention will become commercially available to patients with scleroderma within 20 years of the initial filing. It is important to understand, therefore, that an inventor's patent does not indicate that a product or service is or will be commercially available to patients with scleroderma. The patent implies only that the inventor has "the right to exclude others from making, using, offering for sale, or selling" the invention in the United States. While this relates to U.S. patents, similar rules govern foreign patents.

In this chapter, we show you how to locate information on patents and their inventors. If you find a patent that is particularly interesting to you, contact the inventor or the assignee for further information.

---

[25]Adapted from The U. S. Patent and Trademark Office:
http://www.uspto.gov/web/offices/pac/doc/general/whatis.htm.

Patents on Scleroderma

By performing a patent search focusing on scleroderma, you can obtain information such as the title of the invention, the names of the inventor(s), the assignee(s) or the company that owns or controls the patent, a short abstract that summarizes the patent, and a few excerpts from the description of the patent. The abstract of a patent tends to be more technical in nature, while the description is often written for the public. Full patent descriptions contain much more information than is presented here (e.g. claims, references, figures, diagrams, etc.). We will tell you how to obtain this information later in the chapter. The following is an example of the type of information that you can expect to obtain from a patent search on scleroderma:

- **Diagnostic methods for screening patients for scleroderma**

  Inventor(s): Doxsey; Stephen J. (Worcester, MA)

  Assignee(s): University of Massachusetts (Boston, MA)

  Patent Number: 5,861,260

  Date filed: November 5, 1996

  Abstract: Disclosed are diagnostic methods for screening a patient for sclerotic disease. One diagnostic method includes obtaining a biological sample from the patient; obtaining a substantially pure CP140 polypeptide fragment; contacting the sample with the CP140 polypeptide; and detecting patient autoantibody:CP140 complexes as an indication of the presence of sclerotic disease in the patient. Other methods of screening patients for scleroderma are also described.

  Excerpt(s): The invention relates to cell biology, autoimmune disorders, and diagnosis of scleroderma. ... Scleroderma, or systemic sclerosis, is characterized by deposition of fibrous connective tissue in the skin, and often in many other organ systems. It may be accompanied by vascular lesions, especially in the skin, lungs, and kidneys. The course of this disease is variable, but it is usually slowly progressive. Scleroderma may be limited in scope and compatible with a normal life span. Systemic involvement, however, can be fatal. ... Scleroderma is classified as diffuse or limited, on the basis of the extent of skin and internal organ involvement. The diffuse form is characterized by thickening and fibrosis of skin over the proximal extremities and trunk. The heart, lungs, kidneys, and gastrointestinal tract below the esophagus are often involved. Limited scleroderma is characterized by cutaneous involvement of the hands and face. Visceral involvement occurs less commonly. The limited form has a better prognosis than the diffuse form, except when pulmonary hypertension is present.

Web site: http://www.delphion.com/details?pn=US05861260__

- **Diagnosis of scleroderma and related diseases**

Inventor(s): Nelson; J. Lee (Seattle, WA)

Assignee(s): Fred Hutchinson Cancer Research Center (Seattle, WA)

Patent Number: 5,759,766

Date filed: July 19, 1996

Abstract: Allogeneic cells are removed from an individual predisposed to or suffering from scleroderma or related diseases, thereby treating the disease and inhibiting or preventing its recurrence. Allogeneic cells are identified in the individual and treatment tailored to remove such cells, in vivo or ex vivo, from the individual by cell separation or cytotoxic agents.

Excerpt(s): Women are more frequently affected by autoimmune diseases (Rose et al., Immunol. Today 14:426-430 (1993)) than men, including both rheumatologic and non-rheumatologic autoimmune disorders. Female to male ratios of greater than 5 to 1 have been reported, for example, for scleroderma, systemic lupus erythematosus, Sjogren's syndrome, Hashimoto's thyroiditis, and primary biliary cirrhosis (Silman, Ann. Rheum. Dis. 50(4):887-893 (1991); Hochberg, Arthritis Rheum. 28:80-86 (1985); Kelly et al., Brit. J. Rheumatol. 30:437-442 (1991); Furszyfer et al., Mayo Clin. Proc. 45:586-596 (1970); and Danielsson et al., Heptology 11:458-464 (1990)). Numerous studies have investigated sex hormones and autoimmunity, particularly in animal models of autoimmune disease, and some have demonstrated immunomodulatory effects of sex steroids (Grossman, Science 227:257-261 (1985); and Lahita, Ann. NY Acad. Sci. 658:278-287 (1993)). Perhaps as a result of these studies, the female predilection for autoimmune disease has sometimes been attributed to female/male differences in sex hormones. However, convincing correlations of studies in animal models with human autoimmune diseases have been limited and at least three additional observations argue against this assumption. These include the age-specific incidence patterns of different autoimmune diseases in women, contrasting effects of exogenous sex steroid administration, and contrasting effects of pregnancy. ... Scleroderma is a disease with female/male ratios as high as 14:1, and in which the peak age-specific incidence for women is 35-54, i.e. after child bearing years (Silman, Ann. Rheum. Dis. 50(4):887-893 (1991)). Scleroderma, also referred to as progressive systemic scleroderma, is characterized by diffuse fibrosis, degenerative changes, and vascular abnormalities in the skin, articular structures, and internal organs, especially the esophagus, intestinal tract, thyroid, lung, heart and kidney. The disease varies in severity and progression, with its features ranging from generalized cutaneous thickening with rapidly progressive and often fatal visceral involvement, to a form distinguished by restricted skin involvement and prolonged passage of time before full manifestation of internal disease. Scleroderma bears a striking resemblance to graft-versus-host disease that occurs in some patients after bone marrow transplantation (Chosidow et al., J. Am. Acad. Dermatol 26:49-55 (1992); Claman, Curr. Opin. Rheumatol 2:929-931 (1990); Majoor et al., J. Rheumatol 15:1339-1345 (1988); Graham-Brown et al., Clin. Exp. Dermatol 8:531-538 (1983); Furst et al., Arthritis Rheum. 22:904-910 (1979); and Lawley et al., Ann Int. Med. 87:707-709 (1977)). Treatment is primarily immunosuppressive in nature, e.g., corticosteroids, colchicine or other immunosuppressive agents, which may be used in conjunction with agents which provide symptomatic relief. Prognosis is poor if cardiac, pulmonary or renal manifestations are present at time of diagnosis. ... What is urgently needed is a means for treating individuals predisposed to or suffering from scleroderma or related diseases. Based on an understanding of the events which are associated with development of the disease, new methods for therapeutic or prophylactic intervention in the disease process can be devised. Quite surprisingly, the present invention addresses this and other related needs.

Web site: http://www.delphion.com/details?pn=US05759766__

Patent Applications on Scleroderma

As of December 2000, U.S. patent applications are open to public viewing.[26] Applications are patent requests which have yet to be granted (the process to achieve a patent can take several years).

Keeping Current

In order to stay informed about patents and patent applications dealing with scleroderma, you can access the U.S. Patent Office archive via the Internet at no cost to you. This archive is available at the following Web address:

---

[26] This has been a common practice outside the United States prior to December 2000.

http://www.uspto.gov/main/patents.htm. Under "Services," click on "Search Patents." You will see two broad options: (1) Patent Grants, and (2) Patent Applications. To see a list of granted patents, perform the following steps: Under "Patent Grants," click "Quick Search." Then, type "scleroderma" (or synonyms) into the "Term 1" box. After clicking on the search button, scroll down to see the various patents which have been granted to date on scleroderma. You can also use this procedure to view pending patent applications concerning scleroderma. Simply go back to the following Web address: **http://www.uspto.gov/main/patents.htm**. Under "Services," click on "Search Patents." Select "Quick Search" under "Patent Applications." Then proceed with the steps listed above.

Vocabulary Builder

Biliary: Pertaining to the bile, to the bile ducts, or to the gallbladder. [EU]

Cirrhosis: Liver disease characterized pathologically by loss of the normal microscopic lobular architecture, with fibrosis and nodular regeneration. The term is sometimes used to refer to chronic interstitial inflammation of any organ. [EU]

Cytotoxic: Pertaining to or exhibiting cytotoxicity. [EU]

Exogenous: Developed or originating outside the organism, as exogenous disease. [EU]

Recurrence: The return of a sign, symptom, or disease after a remission. [NIH]

CHAPTER 6. BOOKS ON SCLERODERMA

Overview

This chapter provides bibliographic book references relating to scleroderma. You have many options to locate books on scleroderma. The simplest method is to go to your local bookseller and inquire about titles that they have in stock or can special order for you. Some patients, however, feel uncomfortable approaching their local booksellers and prefer online sources (e.g. **www.amazon.com** and **www.bn.com**). In addition to online booksellers, excellent sources for book titles on scleroderma include the Combined Health Information Database and the National Library of Medicine. Once you have found a title that interests you, visit your local public or medical library to see if it is available for loan.

Book Summaries: Federal Agencies

The Combined Health Information Database collects various book abstracts from a variety of healthcare institutions and federal agencies. To access these summaries, go to **http://chid.nih.gov/detail/detail.html**. You will need to use the "Detailed Search" option. To find book summaries, use the drop boxes at the bottom of the search page where "You may refine your search by." Select the dates and language you prefer. For the format option, select "Monograph/Book." Now type "scleroderma" (or synonyms) into the "For these words:" box. You will only receive results on books. You should check back periodically with this database which is updated every 3 months. The following is a typical result when searching for books on scleroderma:

- **Your Child With Arthritis: A Family Guide for Caregiving**

  Source: Baltimore, MD: The Johns Hopkins University Press. 1996. 339 p.

Contact: Johns Hopkins University Press, 2715 North Charles Street, Baltimore, MD 21218-4319.

Summary: This book for health professionals, families of children with rheumatic illnesses, and older patients provides them with information on dealing with a rheumatic illness. Rheumatic diseases of childhood are described, including juvenile rheumatoid arthritis, juvenile spondyloarthropathy syndromes, systemic lupus erythematosus, dermatomyositis, scleroderma, and vasculitis. The description of each of these diseases includes an explanation of how it is diagnosed and treated, the possible course of the disease, and possible outcomes. Diagnostic laboratory tests and procedures are explained, and medications, physical and occupational therapy, and other treatments are discussed. In addition, the book covers the topics of selecting a physician, developing a positive physician-patient relationship, monitoring a child's progress, creating a positive school environment, financing health care, and coping with the impact of illness on the family. Sample forms are provided to help parents track their child's progress, maintain detailed medical records, and organize pertinent information. A glossary is also included. Appendices present a sample clinic guide and identify other sources of help. 68 references, 1 figure, and 3 tables.

- **Diseases of the Oral Mucosa and the Lips**

Source: Orlando, FL: W.B. Saunders Company. 1993. 389 p.

Contact: Available from W.B. Saunders Company. Order Fulfillment, 6277 Sea Harbor Drive, Orlando, FL 32887-4430. (800) 545-2522 (individuals) or (800) 782-4479 (schools); Fax (800) 874-6418 or (407) 352-3445; http://www.wbsaunders.com. Price: $99.00 plus shipping and handling. ISBN: 0721640397.

Summary: This book is a clinically oriented atlas and text covering the symptoms and diseases of the oral mucosa and perioral skin. The authors focus on the essential aspects of each illness, concentrating on the clinical features that are important in the differential diagnosis. The authors include not only diseases confined to the oral mucosa but also those oral problems that may be signs of accompanying cutaneous (skin) or systemic diseases. Sixty-seven chapters are presented in three sections: the normal oral mucosa, general aspects of oral pathology, and diseases of the oral mucosa and the lips. Specific topics are inflammation of the lips, acquired diseases of the tongue, gingival hyperplasia, enlargement of the parotid gland, aphthous ulcers (stomatitis), pyostomatitis vegetans, disorders of pigmentation, urticaria and angioedema, psoriasis, Reiter's syndrome, lichen planus, graft-versus-host disease, rosacea, perioral dermatitis, erythema multiforme, acute febrile neutrophilic dermatosis

(Sweet's syndrome), vesicular and bullous autoimmune diseases, desquamative gingivitis, necrotizing sialometaplasia, oral mucosal hemorrhage, viral diseases, bacterial diseases, fungal diseases, protozoal and parasitic diseases, mechanical damage, trauma, allergic and toxic contact stomatitis, occupational diseases of the oral mucosa, drug reactions and side effects, morphea and scleroderma, lichen sclerosus et atrophicus, dermatomyositis, lupus erythematosus, Sjogren's syndrome, polyarteritis nodosa, giant cell arteritis, plasma cell gingivitis, oral submucous fibrosis, halitosis, xerostomia, sialorrhea, self-induced mucosal injuries, benign granulomatous processes, malignant granulomatoses, heterotopias and congenital malformations, genodermatoses and congenital syndromes, benign and malignant tumors, actinic keratosis, leukoplakia, paraneoplastic disorders, and oral signs of hematologic, nutritional, metabolic, and endocrine disorders. Each chapter includes full-color photographs and references are provided in individual sections. A subject index concludes the volume. (AA-M).

- **Systemic Sclerosis**

  Source: Baltimore, MD: Williams and Wilkins. 1996. 679 p.

  Contact: Available from Williams and Wilkins, Special Sales Department. (800) 358-3583.

  Summary: This textbook for health professionals provides them with up-to-date information on systemic sclerosis (SSc). Part one presents information on the history, epidemiology, demographics, genetic aspects, classification, prognosis, and differential diagnosis of SSc. Localized scleroderma is described, and the role of environmental factors in scleroderma and pseudoscleroderma is examined. Part two explores the pathogenesis of scleroderma, focusing on cellular aspects, vascular involvement, serologic correlates, environmental aspects, immune aspects, and animal models of systemic sclerosis. Part three discusses pulmonary, cardiac, peripheral vascular, skin, musculoskeletal, renal, nervous system, and gastrointestinal involvement in SSc. In addition, the association between Sjogren's syndrome and SSc is examined, and the sexual and psychosocial aspects of SSc are explored. Part four addresses issues related to designing trials of therapeutic interventions in SSc and describes the use of disease modifying drugs, unproven remedies, surgery, and occupational and physical therapy in treating SSc. Part five examines ancillary and supportive care for SSc patients and lists available resources. Appendices list resources for devices and modalities, Scleroderma Foundation Offices, and products and services. Numerous references, numerous figures, numerous tables, and 15 color plates.

- **Kidney in Collagen-Vascular Diseases**

  Source: New York, NY: Raven Press, Ltd. 1993. 258 p.

  Contact: Available from Raven Press. 1185 Avenue of the Americas, Dept. 5B, New York, NY 10036. (800) 777-2836 or (212) 930-9500. Fax (212) 869-3495. Price: $107.50 plus $4.95 shipping and handling (as of 1995). ISBN: 0781700213.

  Summary: This book brings together current thinking about the effects of various collagen-vascular diseases on the kidney and the diagnostic and therapeutic procedures currently available. These diseases comprise a heterogeneous group of acute and chronic inflammatory, degenerative, and sclerosing processes in the connective tissues and the walls of blood vessels. Eleven chapters cover experimental animal models of systemic lupus erythematosus (SLE); immunology and pathogenesis; lupus-like syndrome; SLE in humans; scleroderma (systemic sclerosis); rheumatoid arthritis and ankylosing spondylitis; mixed connective tissue disease; Sjogren's syndrome; systemic vasculitis; and other collagen diseases, including relapsing polychondritis, acute rheumatic fever, and polymyositis/dermatomyositis. Each chapter includes numerous references and a subject index concludes the volume.

Book Summaries: Online Booksellers

Commercial Internet-based booksellers, such as Amazon.com and Barnes & Noble.com, offer summaries which have been supplied by each title's publisher. Some summaries also include customer reviews. Your local bookseller may have access to in-house and commercial databases that index all published books (e.g. Books in Print®). The following have been recently listed with online booksellers as relating to scleroderma (sorted alphabetically by title; follow the hyperlink to view more details at Amazon.com):

- **An Intimate Account: My Twenty-Five Year Battle Before and After the Diagnosis of Scleroderma and Periarthritis** by Victoria E. Murray Pruitt (2000); ISBN: 0533130921;
  http://www.amazon.com/exec/obidos/ASIN/0533130921/icongroupinterna

- **Connective Tissue Diseases: Lupus, Scleroderma and Rheumatoid Arthritis** by Susan Brown (Editor), Robert P. Sundel (Editor) (1994); ISBN: 187977206X;

http://www.amazon.com/exec/obidos/ASIN/187977206X/icongroupi nterna

- **Scleroderma (Progressive Systemic Sclerosis)** by Alfred John Barnett; ISBN: 0398029555; http://www.amazon.com/exec/obidos/ASIN/0398029555/icongroupin terna

- **Scleroderma and pseudoscleroderma** by Stefania Jabłoânska; ISBN: 0879331402; http://www.amazon.com/exec/obidos/ASIN/0879331402/icongroupin terna

- **Scleroderma: A New Role For Patients and Families** by Michael Brown; ISBN: 0971752400; http://www.amazon.com/exec/obidos/ASIN/0971752400/icongroupin terna

- **Scleroderma: Caring for Your Hands & Feet** by Jeanne L. Melvin, Bradley O. Pomeroy (Illustrator) (1994); ISBN: 1569000069; http://www.amazon.com/exec/obidos/ASIN/1569000069/icongroupin terna

- **Scleroderma: The Proven Therapy That Can Save Your Life** by Henry Scammell (1998); ISBN: 0871318423; http://www.amazon.com/exec/obidos/ASIN/0871318423/icongroupin terna

- **Successful Living with Scleroderma** by Robert H. Phillips; ISBN: 1888614102; http://www.amazon.com/exec/obidos/ASIN/1888614102/icongroupin terna

- **Systemic Sclerosis: Scleroderma** by Malcolm I. Jayson (Editor), Carol M. Black (Editor); ISBN: 0471908460; http://www.amazon.com/exec/obidos/ASIN/0471908460/icongroupin terna

- **The Scleroderma Book: A Guide for Patients and Families** by Maureen D. Mayes; ISBN: 0195115074; http://www.amazon.com/exec/obidos/ASIN/0195115074/icongroupin terna

The National Library of Medicine Book Index

The National Library of Medicine at the National Institutes of Health has a massive database of books published on healthcare and biomedicine. Go to the following Internet site, **http://locatorplus.gov/**, and then select "Search LOCATORplus." Once you are in the search area, simply type "scleroderma" (or synonyms) into the search box, and select "books only." From there, results can be sorted by publication date, author, or relevance. The following was recently catalogued by the National Library of Medicine.[27]

- **Autoimmune diseases of the skin: pathogenesis, diagnosis, management.** Author: Michael Hertl (ed.); Year: 2001; Wien; New York: Springer, c2001; ISBN: 3211835989 (alk. paper)
  http://www.amazon.com/exec/obidos/ASIN/3211835989/icongroupin terna

- **Collagen diseases: including systemic lupus erythematosus, polyarteritis, dermatomyositis, systemic scleroderma, thrombotic thrombocytopenic purpura.** Author: John H. Talbott and R. Moleres Ferrandis; Year: 1956; New York: Grune & Stratton, 1956

- **Connective tissue diseases: lupus, scleroderma, and rheumatoid arthritis.** Author: medical consultant, Robert P. Sundel; contributor, Susan Brown; editor, Joan Schulman; Year: 1995; Miami, FL (P.O. Box 163200 Miami 3311-63200): Health Studies Institute, c1995

- **Control mechanisms in scleroderma: Fulmer Grange Conference Centre, Flumer, Slough, Berkshire, UK, Thursday 23 and Friday 24th April 1987.** Author: sponsored by Smith, Kline and French Laboratories Limited; organized by C.M. Black; Year: 1988; [London]: The Council, [1988?]

- **Dental manifestations of acrosclerosis and diffuse scleroderma.** Author: Rugeley, Robert Austin; Year: 1955; [Minneapolis] 1955

- **Dermatomyositis, with special reference to the differential diagnosis of scleroderma.** Author: Brock, William George, 1905-; Year: 1933; [Minneapolis] 1933

- **Heart in progressive systemic sclerosis; a clinical pathologic study.** Author: Rottenberg, Everett Newton, 1927-; Year: 1957; [Minneapolis] 1957

---

[27] In addition to LOCATORPlus, in collaboration with authors and publishers, the National Center for Biotechnology Information (NCBI) is adapting biomedical books for the Web. The books may be accessed in two ways: (1) by searching directly using any search term or phrase (in the same way as the bibliographic database PubMed), or (2) by following the links to PubMed abstracts. Each PubMed abstract has a "Books" button that displays a facsimile of the abstract in which some phrases are hypertext links. These phrases are also found in the books available at NCBI. Click on hyperlinked results in the list of books in which the phrase is found. Currently, the majority of the links are between the books and PubMed. In the future, more links will be created between the books and other types of information, such as gene and protein sequences and macromolecular structures. See **http://www.ncbi.nlm.nih.gov/entrez/query.fcgi?db=Books.**

- **Hemiatrophy associated with scleroderma and other conditions.** Author: Christianson, Herbert Bernard, 1915-; Year: 1956; [Minneapolis] 1956

- **Immunological studies in Raynaud's phenomenon.** Author: door Jan van der Meulen; Year: 1979; [Groningen?: s.n.], 1979

- **Localized scleroderma (morphoea): clinical, physiological, biochemical and ultrastructural studies with particular reference to quantitation of scleroderma.** Author: by Jørgen Serup; Year: 1986; Stockholm, Sweden: Distributed by Almqvist & Wiksell Periodical Co., [1986]; ISBN: 8798211811 (pbk.)

- **Lung in scleroderma; a clinical-pathological study.** Author: Weaver, Arthur Lawrence, 1936-; Year: 1966; [Minneapolis] 1966

- **Many faces of scleroderma.** Author: J. Donald Smiley; Year: 1992; [Dallas: University of Texas Southwestern Medical Center at Dallas, Parkland Memorial Hospital, 1992]

- **Patients with connective tissue diseases: lupus, scleroderma, rheumatoid arthritis.** Author: Carroll Cameron; consultants, Larry Garland, Michael haiken, Janine D'Agostino Plavac; Year: 1987; Miami, FL (P.O. Box 164600, Miami, 33116-4600): Health Studies Institute, c1987

- **Proceedings of the Scleroderma Symposium: held at the Barbican Centre, London on 12 and 13 May 1983.** Author: edited by Carol M. Black; Year: 1983; Mundells, Welwyn Garden City, Hertforshire: Smith Kline & French Laboratories, c1983; ISBN: 095032924X

- **Progressive systemic sclerosis, or visceral scleroderma; review of literature and report of cases, by M. L. Orabona and O. Albano.** Author: Orabona, M. L; Year: 1958; Bari, 1958

- **Role of hydroxyproline in scleroderma.** Author: Neldner, Kenneth Herbert, 1927-; Year: 1963; [Minneapolis] 1963

- **Scleroderma (progressive systemic sclerosis).** Author: Barnett, Alfred John; Year: 1974; Springfield, Ill., Thomas [c1974]; ISBN: 0398029555 http://www.amazon.com/exec/obidos/ASIN/0398029555/icongroupin terna

- **Scleroderma and pseudoscleroderma.** Author: edited by Stefania Jablo´nska; Year: 1975; Warsaw: Polish Medical Publishers; Stroudsburg, Pa.: distributed by Dowden, Hutchinson & Ross, c1975; ISBN: 0879331402 http://www.amazon.com/exec/obidos/ASIN/0879331402/icongroupin terna

- **Scleroderma and pseudoscleroderma; systemic scleroderma, morphea, and allied conditions. Contributors: Zdzislaw Askanas [and] Stanislaw**

> **Leszczy´nski.** Author: Jablo´nska, Stefania; Year: 1965; Warsaw, Polish Medical Publishers, 1965

- **Scleroderma of the gastrointestinal tract; a clinical-pathological study.** Author: Treacy, William Laurence, 1932-; Year: 1960; [Minneapolis] 1960

- **Scleroderma.** Author: Sackner, Marvin A., 1932-; Year: 1966; New York, Grune & Stratton, 1966

- **Scleroderma: a twenty year study.** Author: Tuffanelli, Denny Lee, 1929-; Year: 1961; [Minneapolis] 1961

- **Scleroderma; the relationship of calcinosis and the effects of a new chelating agent, EDTA.** Author: Muller, Sigfrid Augustine, 1930-; Year: 1958; [Minneapolis] 1958

- **Study of the joint manifestations in scleroderma.** Author: Clark, John Arnot, 1935-; Year: 1967; [Minneapolis] 1967

- **Systemic sclerosis (scleroderma): based on the proceedings of the International Conferencee on Progressive Systemic Sclerosis held October 20-23, 1981, Austin, Texas.** Author: [edited by] Carol M. Black, Allen R. Myers; Year: 1985; New York: Gower Medical Pub., c1985; ISBN: 0912143088
http://www.amazon.com/exec/obidos/ASIN/0912143088/icongroupin terna

- **Systemic sclerosis: scleroderma.** Author: edited by Malcolm I.V. Jayson, Carol M. Black; Year: 1988; Chichester; New York: Wiley; New York, NY, USA: Distributed in the U.S.A., Canada, and Japan by Liss, c1988; ISBN: 0471908460
http://www.amazon.com/exec/obidos/ASIN/0471908460/icongroupin terna

Chapters on Scleroderma

Frequently, scleroderma will be discussed within a book, perhaps within a specific chapter. In order to find chapters that are specifically dealing with scleroderma, an excellent source of abstracts is the Combined Health Information Database. You will need to limit your search to book chapters and scleroderma using the "Detailed Search" option. Go directly to the following hyperlink: **http://chid.nih.gov/detail/detail.html**. To find book chapters, use the drop boxes at the bottom of the search page where "You may refine your search by." Select the dates and language you prefer, and the format option "Book Chapter." By making these selections and typing in "scleroderma" (or synonyms) into the "For these words:" box, you will only receive results on chapters in books. The following is a typical result when searching for book chapters on scleroderma:

- **Chapter 20: Systemic Sclerosis and Related Syndromes**

  Source: in Klippel, J.H., et al., eds. Primer on the Rheumatic Diseases. 11th ed. Atlanta, GA: Arthritis Foundation. 1997. p. 263-275.

  Contact: Available from Arthritis Foundation. P.O. Box 1616, Alpharetta, GA 30009-1616. (800) 207-8633. Fax (credit card orders only) (770) 442-9742. Website: www.arthritis.org. Price: $39.95 plus shipping and handling. ISBN: 0912423161.

  Summary: This chapter provides health professionals with information on the epidemiology, pathology, pathogenesis, clinical features, and treatment of systemic sclerosis and related syndromes. Scleroderma encompasses both disease restricted to the skin and disease with internal organ involvement. The latter form, which is known as diffuse scleroderma or systemic sclerosis, is an acquired, noncontagious, rare disease that occurs worldwide. Although the etiology of systemic sclerosis is unknown, susceptibility appears to be controlled by a complex interaction between environmental influences such as inhaled or ingested chemicals and viruses, as well as genetic factors such as gender and nongenetic host factors such as age. Its clinical course is influenced by genetic factors. Pathological features include widespread small vessel vasculopathy and fibrosis. The immune system, multiple cytokines, endothelial cell activity, and fibroblast abnormalities are likely involved in the pathogenesis of systemic sclerosis. The initial symptoms are typically nonspecific and include Raynaud's phenomenon, lack of energy or fatigue, and musculoskeletal complaints. Most patients who have limited scleroderma gradually develop features of the CREST syndrome of calcinosis, Raynaud's phenomenon, esophageal dysmotility, sclerodactyly, and telangiectasia. The chapter discusses Raynaud's phenomenon and skin, musculoskeletal, pulmonary, gastrointestinal, cardiac, and renal manifestations of scleroderma. In addition, the chapter describes scleroderma like disorders, including localized scleroderma, environmentally associated disorders, diffuse fasciitis with eosinophilia, and epidemic scleroderma like disorders. The final topic is the treatment of systemic sclerosis with disease modifying drugs and the management of various organ system problems. 10 figures, 3 tables, and 52 references.

- **History of Scleroderma**

  Source: in Clements, P.J.; Furst, D.E., Eds. Systemic Sclerosis. Baltimore, MD: Williams and Wilkins. 1996. p. 3-22.

Contact: Available from Williams and Wilkins, Special Sales Department. (800) 358-3583.

Summary: This chapter for health professionals presents an overview of the history of scleroderma. Possible early cases of scleroderma are identified. Descriptions of scleroderma in the nineteenth century are highlighted. Subdivisions of types of scleroderma are discussed, focusing on systemic sclerosis (SSc) and morphea. Subdivisions of SSc are examined. Descriptions of the involvement of the skin, joints, blood vessels, alimentary tract, lungs, heart, and kidneys are presented. The concept of scleroderma as a systemic disease is discussed. Research on the nature of scleroderma is highlighted, focusing on investigations of scleroderma as a connective tissue disease, a vascular disease, and an autoimmune disease. Views on the causes of scleroderma are presented. In addition, types of therapies that have been used to treat scleroderma are described. 121 references.

- **Scleroderma and Pseudoscleroderma: Environmental Exposure**

  Source: in Clements, P.J.; Furst, D.E., Eds. Systemic Sclerosis. Baltimore, MD: Williams and Wilkins. 1996. p. 81-98.

  Contact: Available from Williams and Wilkins, Special Sales Department. (800) 358-3583.

  Summary: This chapter for health professionals focuses on the association between scleroderma or scleroderma-like conditions and various chemical and environmental exposures. Data on the association between scleroderma and silica and silicone are presented. The causes, clinical features, and treatment of toxic oil syndrome, eosinophilia-myalgia syndrome, and vinyl chloride disease are discussed. The role of organic solvents, amines, bleomycin, and pentazocine in inducing scleroderma or scleroderma-like conditions is examined. Although some of these environmentally linked conditions differ from idiopathic scleroderma, they all tend to produce skin inflammation and fibrosis of the skin and subcutaneous tissue. 144 references, 3 figures, and 2 tables.

- **Differential Diagnosis of Scleroderma-like Disorders**

  Source: in Clements, P.J.; Furst, D.E., Eds. Systemic Sclerosis. Baltimore, MD: Williams and Wilkins. 1996. p. 99-120.

  Contact: Available from Williams and Wilkins, Special Sales Department. (800) 358-3583.

  Summary: This chapter for health professionals focuses on the differential diagnosis of scleroderma-like disorders. These disorders include scleredema, scleredema associated with paraproteinemia or myeloma, scleromyxedema, scleroderma-like lesions in endocrine disorders, Werner's syndrome, progeria, sclerodermiform neonatal progeria, restrictive dermopathy, sclerodermiform chronic graft-versus-host disease, and scleroderma-like changes of porphyria cutanea tarda. Other disorders include scleroderma-like lesions in phenylketonuria, congenital fascial dystrophy, scleroderma-like changes induced by bleomycin, scleroderma-like plaques after vitamin K injection, progressive facial hemiatrophy, fibroblastic rheumatism, localized lipoatrophies, lichen sclerosus et atrophicus, sclerodermiform variety of acrodermatitis chronica atrophicans, and atrophoderma Pasini- pierini. Most of these disorders are discussed in terms of their clinical features, pathology and pathophysiology, differential diagnosis, and treatment. 115 references and 10 figures.

- **Pathogenesis of Scleroderma: Cellular Aspects**

  Source: in Clements, P.J.; Furst, D.E., Eds. Systemic Sclerosis. Baltimore, MD: Williams and Wilkins. 1996. p. 123-152.

  Contact: Available from Williams and Wilkins, Special Sales Department. (800) 358-3583.

  Summary: This chapter for health professionals explores the cellular aspects of the pathogenesis of systemic sclerosis (SSc). Current knowledge about SSc fibroblast morphology and fibroblast function in SSc is reviewed. The structure and regulation of the type I collagen genes are described. Immune activation and the involvement of cytokines in the pathogenesis of fibrosis in SSc are discussed. The modulation of connective tissue accumulation by cytokines is examined. The effect of specific cytokines on collagen metabolism is reviewed, focusing on interferons, tumor necrosis factors, interleukin-1, other interleukins, and transforming growth factor-beta (TGFB). The role of TGFB in the pathogenesis of SSc and other fibrotic conditions is discussed. The role of platelet-derived growth factor, fibroblast growth factors, epidermal growth factors, prostaglandins, mast cells, and eosinophils in SSc is highlighted. The role of retroviral proteins in the activation of collagen gene expression is examined. The interaction of the extracellular matrix and extracellular signals and their effects on fibroblast connective tissue synthesis are explained. 228 references, 8 figures, and 3 tables.

- **Scleroderma Patient Support Groups and Organizations**

  Source: in Clements, P.J.; Furst, D.E., Eds. Systemic Sclerosis. Baltimore, MD: Williams and Wilkins. 1996. p. 621-632.

Contact: Available from Williams and Wilkins, Special Sales Department. (800) 358-3583.

Summary: This chapter for health professionals describes the Scleroderma Federation and the United Scleroderma Foundation, Inc. The Scleroderma Federation is discussed in terms of its mission, office organization, collaborative funding program, meetings, continuing medical education meetings, public awareness and education efforts, and services. Services include publication of a quarterly newsletter, provision of physician referrals and peer counseling, and maintenance of a resource library. The organization of the United Scleroderma Foundation is described, and its services are highlighted. They include providing support to patients and their families, hosting an annual conference, providing patients and health professionals with educational material, publishing a quarterly newsletter, sponsoring medical workshops, providing physician referrals, advocating for patients, enhancing public awareness, and maintaining resources. Appendices list Scleroderma Foundation Offices and products and services. 1 table.

- **Scleroderma in Childhood**

  Source: in Maddison, P.J.; et al., Eds. Oxford Textbook of Rheumatology. Volume 2. New York, NY: Oxford University Press, Inc. 1993. p. 790-794.

  Contact: Available from Oxford University Press, Inc., New York, NY.

  Summary: This chapter for health professionals presents an overview of scleroderma in children. Clinical types of childhood scleroderma are identified. The clinical features of the variants of localized scleroderma are described, including the features of morphoea, linear scleroderma, and en coup de sabre. The features of limited cutaneous systemic sclerosis and diffuse cutaneous systemic sclerosis, two clinical variants of systemic scleroderma, are highlighted. Laboratory abnormalities found in children with scleroderma are discussed. Options for treating childhood scleroderma are presented, including practical measures, physiotherapy, occupational therapy, and drug therapy. The outcome of childhood scleroderma is considered. In addition, scleroderma-like conditions in childhood are identified. 18 references and 5 figures.

- **Morphea and Scleroderma**

  Source: in Bork, K., et al. Diseases of the Oral Mucosa and the Lips. Orlando, FL: W.B. Saunders Company. 1993. p. 204-210.

  Contact: Available from W.B. Saunders Company. Order Fulfillment, 6277 Sea Harbor Drive, Orlando, FL 32887-4430. (800) 545-2522 (individuals) or (800) 782-4479 (schools); Fax (800) 874-6418 or (407) 352-

3445; http://www.wbsaunders.com. Price: $99.00 plus shipping and handling. ISBN: 0721640397.

Summary: This chapter, from a textbook on diseases of the oral mucosa and the lips, discusses morphea and scleroderma, two distinct clinical disorders with an almost identical histologic appearance. Morphea is generally localized and limited to the skin. Scleroderma or progressive systemic sclerosis (PSS) is a wide-spread systemic, often fatal disorder involving the lungs, heart, kidneys, and many other organs. In the skin, both disorders show marked dermal thickening. The chapter also discusses facial hemiatrophy. For each topic, the authors describe the clinical features and present brief therapeutic recommendations. Full-color photographs illustrate the chapter; references are provided for some sections. 15 figures. 26 references. (AA-M).

General Home References

In addition to references for scleroderma, you may want a general home medical guide that spans all aspects of home healthcare. The following list is a recent sample of such guides (sorted alphabetically by title; hyperlinks provide rankings, information, and reviews at Amazon.com):

- **Encyclopedia of Skin and Skin Disorders (The Facts on File Library of Health and Living)** by Carol Turkington, Jeffrey S. Dover; Hardcover - 448 pages, 2nd edition (June 2002), Facts on File, Inc.; ISBN: 0816047766; **http://www.amazon.com/exec/obidos/ASIN/0816047766/icongroupinterna**

- **Your Skin from A to Z** by Jerome Z. Litt, M.D.; Paperback (March 2002), Barricade Books; ISBN: 1569802165; **http://www.amazon.com/exec/obidos/ASIN/1569802165/icongroupinterna**

- **American College of Physicians Complete Home Medical Guide (with Interactive Human Anatomy CD-ROM)** by David R. Goldmann (Editor), American College of Physicians; Hardcover - 1104 pages, Book & CD-Rom edition (1999), DK Publishing; ISBN: 0789444127; **http://www.amazon.com/exec/obidos/ASIN/0789444127/icongroupinterna**

- **The American Medical Association Guide to Home Caregiving** by the American Medical Association (Editor); Paperback - 256 pages 1 edition (2001), John Wiley & Sons; ISBN: 0471414093; **http://www.amazon.com/exec/obidos/ASIN/0471414093/icongroupinterna**

- **Anatomica : The Complete Home Medical Reference** by Peter Forrestal (Editor); Hardcover (2000), Book Sales; ISBN: 1740480309; http://www.amazon.com/exec/obidos/ASIN/1740480309/icongroupinterna

- **The HarperCollins Illustrated Medical Dictionary : The Complete Home Medical Dictionary** by Ida G. Dox, et al; Paperback - 656 pages 4th edition (2001), Harper Resource; ISBN: 0062736469; http://www.amazon.com/exec/obidos/ASIN/0062736469/icongroupinterna

- **Mayo Clinic Guide to Self-Care: Answers for Everyday Health Problems** by Philip Hagen, M.D. (Editor), et al; Paperback - 279 pages, 2nd edition (December 15, 1999), Kensington Publishing Corp.; ISBN: 0962786578; http://www.amazon.com/exec/obidos/ASIN/0962786578/icongroupinterna

- **The Merck Manual of Medical Information : Home Edition (Merck Manual of Medical Information Home Edition (Trade Paper)** by Robert Berkow (Editor), Mark H. Beers, M.D. (Editor); Paperback - 1536 pages (2000), Pocket Books; ISBN: 0671027263; http://www.amazon.com/exec/obidos/ASIN/0671027263/icongroupinterna

Vocabulary Builder

Acrodermatitis: Inflammation involving the skin of the extremities, especially the hands and feet. Several forms are known, some idiopathic and some hereditary. The infantile form is called Gianotti-Crosti syndrome. [NIH]

Alimentary: Pertaining to food or nutritive material, or to the organs of digestion. [EU]

Angioedema: A vascular reaction involving the deep dermis or subcutaneous or submucal tissues, representing localized edema caused by dilatation and increased permeability of the capillaries, and characterized by development of giant wheals. [EU]

Dermatosis: Any skin disease, especially one not characterized by inflammation. [EU]

Dystrophy: Any disorder arising from defective or faulty nutrition, especially the muscular dystrophies. [EU]

Eosinophilia: The formation and accumulation of an abnormally large number of eosinophils in the blood. [EU]

Eosinophils: Granular leukocytes with a nucleus that usually has two lobes connected by a slender thread of chromatin, and cytoplasm containing coarse, round granules that are uniform in size and stainable by eosin. [NIH]

Epidemic: Occurring suddenly in numbers clearly in excess of normal expectancy; said especially of infectious diseases but applied also to any disease, injury, or other health-related event occurring in such outbreaks. [EU]

Epidermal: Pertaining to or resembling epidermis. Called also epidermic or epidermoid. [EU]

Febrile: Pertaining to or characterized by fever. [EU]

Gingivitis: Inflammation of the gingivae. Gingivitis associated with bony changes is referred to as periodontitis. Called also oulitis and ulitis. [EU]

Halitosis: An offensive, foul breath odor resulting from a variety of causes such as poor oral hygiene, dental or oral infections, or the ingestion of certain foods. [NIH]

Hemorrhage: Bleeding or escape of blood from a vessel. [NIH]

Hobbies: Leisure activities engaged in for pleasure. [NIH]

Hydroxyproline: A hydroxylated form of the imino acid proline. A deficiency in ascorbic acid can result in impaired hydroxyproline formation. [NIH]

Hyperplasia: The abnormal multiplication or increase in the number of normal cells in normal arrangement in a tissue. [EU]

Interferons: Proteins secreted by vertebrate cells in response to a wide variety of inducers. They confer resistance against many different viruses, inhibit proliferation of normal and malignant cells, impede multiplication of intracellular parasites, enhance macrophage and granulocyte phagocytosis, augment natural killer cell activity, and show several other immunomodulatory functions. [NIH]

Interleukins: Soluble factors which stimulate growth-related activities of leukocytes as well as other cell types. They enhance cell proliferation and differentiation, DNA synthesis, secretion of other biologically active molecules and responses to immune and inflammatory stimuli. [NIH]

Keratosis: Any horny growth such as a wart or callus. [NIH]

Malformation: A morphologic defect resulting from an intrinsically abnormal developmental process. [EU]

Microscopy: The application of microscope magnification to the study of materials that cannot be properly seen by the unaided eye. [NIH]

Mucosa: A mucous membrane, or tunica mucosa. [EU]

Myalgia: Pain in a muscle or muscles. [EU]

Myeloma: A tumour composed of cells of the type normally found in the bone marrow. [EU]

Necrosis: The sum of the morphological changes indicative of cell death and caused by the progressive degradative action of enzymes; it may affect groups of cells or part of a structure or an organ. [EU]

Neonatal: Pertaining to the first four weeks after birth. [EU]

Parasitic: Pertaining to, of the nature of, or caused by a parasite. [EU]

Perioral: Situated or occurring around the mouth. [EU]

Progeria: An abnormal congenital condition characterized by premature aging in children, where all the changes of cell senescence occur. It is manifested by premature greying, hair loss, hearing loss, cataracts, arthritis,osteoporosis, diabetes mellitus, atrophy of subcutaneous fat, skeletal hypoplasia, and accelerated atherosclerosis. Many affected individuals develop malignant tumors, especially sarcomas. [NIH]

Purpura: Purplish or brownish red discoloration, easily visible through the epidermis, caused by hemorrhage into the tissues. [NIH]

Sialorrhea: Increased salivary flow. [NIH]

Spondylitis: Inflammation of the vertebrae. [EU]

Stomatitis: Inflammation of the oral mucosa, due to local or systemic factors which may involve the buccal and labial mucosa, palate, tongue, floor of the mouth, and the gingivae. [EU]

Urticaria: Pathology: a transient condition of the skin, usually caused by an allergic reaction, characterized by pale or reddened irregular, elevated patches and severe itching; hives. [EU]

Vasculitis: Inflammation of a vessel, angiitis. [EU]

Vesicular: 1. composed of or relating to small, saclike bodies. 2. pertaining to or made up of vesicles on the skin. [EU]

Viruses: Minute infectious agents whose genomes are composed of DNA or RNA, but not both. They are characterized by a lack of independent metabolism and the inability to replicate outside living host cells. [NIH]

CHAPTER 7. MULTIMEDIA ON SCLERODERMA

Overview

Information on scleroderma can come in a variety of formats. Among multimedia sources, video productions, slides, audiotapes, and computer databases are often available. In this chapter, we show you how to keep current on multimedia sources of information on scleroderma. We start with sources that have been summarized by federal agencies, and then show you how to find bibliographic information catalogued by the National Library of Medicine. If you see an interesting item, visit your local medical library to check on the availability of the title.

Video Recordings

Most diseases do not have a video dedicated to them. If they do, they are often rather technical in nature. An excellent source of multimedia information on scleroderma is the Combined Health Information Database. You will need to limit your search to "video recording" and "scleroderma" using the "Detailed Search" option. Go directly to the following hyperlink: **http://chid.nih.gov/detail/detail.html**. To find video productions, use the drop boxes at the bottom of the search page where "You may refine your search by." Select the dates and language you prefer, and the format option "Videorecording (videotape, videocassette, etc.)." By making these selections and typing "scleroderma" (or synonyms) into the "For these words:" box, you will only receive results on video productions. The following is a typical result when searching for video recordings on scleroderma:

- **Power of Two**

  Source: Santa Barbara, CA: Scleroderma Research Foundation. (videocassette).

  Contact: Available from Scleroderma Research Foundation. 2320 Bath Street, Suite 307, Santa Barbara, CA 93105. (800) 441-2873 or (805) 563-9133; FAX (805) 563-2402. Price: $6.50.

  Summary: This videorecording portrays the story of Sharon Monsky, who founded the Scleroderma Research Foundation. Ms. Monsky talks about how scleroderma has affected her life, her family, and their activities of daily living. An overview of the unique approach to collaborative research undertaken by the Scleroderma Research Foundation also is provided.

Bibliography: Multimedia on Scleroderma

The National Library of Medicine is a rich source of information on healthcare-related multimedia productions including slides, computer software, and databases. To access the multimedia database, go to the following Web site: **http://locatorplus.gov/.** Select "Search LOCATORplus." Once in the search area, simply type in scleroderma (or synonyms). Then, in the option box provided below the search box, select "Audiovisuals and Computer Files." From there, you can choose to sort results by publication date, author, or relevance. The following multimedia has been indexed on scleroderma. For more information, follow the hyperlink indicated:

- **Cutaneous manifestations of systemic disease.** Source: American Academy of Dermatology, and Institute for Dermatologic Communication and Education; Year: 1973; Format: Slide; [Evanston, Ill.]: The Academy, [1973]

- **Dermatoses and pregnancy.** Source: Stephen I. Katz; Year: 1972; Format: Slide; New York: Medcom, c1972

- **Scleroderma, SLE.** Source: produced by Audio Master; Year: 1988; Format: Sound recording; [Atlanta, Ga.]: American Rheumatism Association, [1988]

- **Scleroderma.** Source: Maria Guttadauria; Year: 1979; Format: Slide; [New York]: Medcom, c1979

Vocabulary Builder

Candidiasis: Infection with a fungus of the genus Candida. It is usually a superficial infection of the moist cutaneous areas of the body, and is generally caused by C. albicans; it most commonly involves the skin (dermatocandidiasis), oral mucous membranes (thrush, def. 1), respiratory tract (bronchocandidiasis), and vagina (vaginitis). Rarely there is a systemic infection or endocarditis. Called also moniliasis, candidosis, oidiomycosis, and formerly blastodendriosis. [EU]

Dehydration: The condition that results from excessive loss of body water. Called also anhydration, deaquation and hypohydration. [EU]

Lubrication: The application of a substance to diminish friction between two surfaces. It may refer to oils, greases, and similar substances for the lubrication of medical equipment but it can be used for the application of substances to tissue to reduce friction, such as lotions for skin and vaginal lubricants. [NIH]

Neural: 1. pertaining to a nerve or to the nerves. 2. situated in the region of the spinal axis, as the neutral arch. [EU]

Sarcoidosis: An idiopathic systemic inflammatory granulomatous disorder comprised of epithelioid and multinucleated giant cells with little necrosis. It usually invades the lungs with fibrosis and may also involve lymph nodes, skin, liver, spleen, eyes, phalangeal bones, and parotid glands. [NIH]

CHAPTER 8. PERIODICALS AND NEWS ON SCLERODERMA

Overview

Keeping up on the news relating to scleroderma can be challenging. Subscribing to targeted periodicals can be an effective way to stay abreast of recent developments on scleroderma. Periodicals include newsletters, magazines, and academic journals.

In this chapter, we suggest a number of news sources and present various periodicals that cover scleroderma beyond and including those which are published by patient associations mentioned earlier. We will first focus on news services, and then on periodicals. News services, press releases, and newsletters generally use more accessible language, so if you do chose to subscribe to one of the more technical periodicals, make sure that it uses language you can easily follow.

News Services & Press Releases

Well before articles show up in newsletters or the popular press, they may appear in the form of a press release or a public relations announcement. One of the simplest ways of tracking press releases on scleroderma is to search the news wires. News wires are used by professional journalists, and have existed since the invention of the telegraph. Today, there are several major "wires" that are used by companies, universities, and other organizations to announce new medical breakthroughs. In the following sample of sources, we will briefly describe how to access each service. These services only post recent news intended for public viewing.

PR Newswire

Perhaps the broadest of the wires is PR Newswire Association, Inc. To access this archive, simply go to **http://www.prnewswire.com**. Below the search box, select the option "The last 30 days." In the search box, type "scleroderma" or synonyms. The search results are shown by order of relevance. When reading these press releases, do not forget that the sponsor of the release may be a company or organization that is trying to sell a particular product or therapy. Their views, therefore, may be biased.

Reuters

The Reuters' Medical News database can be very useful in exploring news archives relating to scleroderma. While some of the listed articles are free to view, others can be purchased for a nominal fee. To access this archive, go to **http://www.reutershealth.com/frame2/arch.html** and search by "scleroderma" (or synonyms). The following was recently listed in this archive for scleroderma:

- **Genetic predisposition to high TGF production seen in systemic sclerosis**
  Source: Reuters Medical News
  Date: August 09, 2002
  http://www.reuters.gov/archive/2002/08/09/professional/links/20020809epid007.html

- **Combination regimen effective against systemic sclerosis lung disease**
  Source: Reuters Industry Breifing
  Date: March 07, 2002
  http://www.reuters.gov/archive/2002/03/07/business/links/20020307clin004.html

- **Nitroglycerine tape improves peripheral circulation in systemic sclerosis**
  Source: Reuters Industry Breifing
  Date: February 06, 2002
  http://www.reuters.gov/archive/2002/02/06/business/links/20020206drgd001.html

- **Interstitial lung disease linked to gastroesophageal reflux in systemic sclerosis**
  Source: Reuters Medical News
  Date: September 12, 2001
  http://www.reuters.gov/archive/2001/09/12/professional/links/20010912clin009.html

- **Scleroderma family registry launched in US**
  Source: Reuters Health eLine
  Date: June 26, 2001
  http://www.reuters.gov/archive/2001/06/26/eline/links/20010626elin030.html

- **Early organ involvement linked to poor outcome in systemic sclerosis**
  Source: Reuters Medical News
  Date: December 26, 2000
  http://www.reuters.gov/archive/2000/12/26/professional/links/20001226clin004.html

- **Greater skin thickness predicts early mortality in patients with systemic sclerosis**
  Source: Reuters Medical News
  Date: December 22, 2000
  http://www.reuters.gov/archive/2000/12/22/professional/links/20001222clin002.html

- **GI involvement common in children with scleroderma and MCTD**
  Source: Reuters Industry Breifing
  Date: December 20, 2000
  http://www.reuters.gov/archive/2000/12/20/business/links/20001220clin001.html

- **Drug combats scleroderma in lab tests**
  Source: Reuters Health eLine
  Date: November 07, 2000
  http://www.reuters.gov/archive/2000/11/07/eline/links/20001107elin020.html

- **Connetics rocked by failure of scleroderma drug**
  Source: Reuters Industry Breifing
  Date: October 09, 2000
  http://www.reuters.gov/archive/2000/10/09/business/links/20001009inds003.html

- **Cellular microchimerism linked to systemic sclerosis**
  Source: Reuters Medical News
  Date: June 22, 2000
  http://www.reuters.gov/archive/2000/06/22/professional/links/20000622scie002.html

- **Relaxin improves skin symptoms of scleroderma**
  Source: Reuters Medical News
  Date: June 06, 2000
  http://www.reuters.gov/archive/2000/06/06/professional/links/20000606clin002.html

- **Pregnancy hormone promising for scleroderma**
  Source: Reuters Health eLine
  Date: June 06, 2000
  http://www.reuters.gov/archive/2000/06/06/eline/links/20000606elin004.html

- **Collgard scleroderma drug gets orphan drug designation**
  Source: Reuters Medical News
  Date: March 13, 2000
  http://www.reuters.gov/archive/2000/03/13/professional/links/20000313rglt003.html

- **Fetal Antimaternal Graft-Vs-Host Reaction Has Role In Scleroderma**
  Source: Reuters Medical News
  Date: April 23, 1998
  http://www.reuters.gov/archive/1998/04/23/professional/links/19980423clin001.html

- **Fetal Cells May Trigger Scleroderma**
  Source: Reuters Health eLine
  Date: April 22, 1998
  http://www.reuters.gov/archive/1998/04/22/eline/links/19980422elin009.html

- **Maternal-Fetal Microchimerism May Be Involved In Scleroderma**
  Source: Reuters Medical News
  Date: February 20, 1998
  http://www.reuters.gov/archive/1998/02/20/professional/links/19980220clin001.html

- **Fetal Cells May Cause Scleroderma**
  Source: Reuters Health eLine
  Date: February 20, 1998
  http://www.reuters.gov/archive/1998/02/20/eline/links/19980220elin003.html

- **Low-Dose Ultraviolet Light Effective Against Localized Scleroderma**
  Source: Reuters Medical News
  Date: February 03, 1998
  http://www.reuters.gov/archive/1998/02/03/professional/links/19980203clin003.html

- **Intestinal Perforations Common In Patients With Scleroderma**
  Source: Reuters Medical News
  Date: April 04, 1997
  http://www.reuters.gov/archive/1997/04/04/professional/links/19970
  404clin007.html

- **Abnormal Metal Status May Underlie Scleroderma Etiology**
  Source: Reuters Medical News
  Date: January 16, 1997
  http://www.reuters.gov/archive/1997/01/16/professional/links/19970
  116scie002.html

- **Early Clues To Scleroderma**
  Source: Reuters Health eLine
  Date: January 14, 1997
  http://www.reuters.gov/archive/1997/01/14/eline/links/19970114elin
  010.html

- **[] - Connective Therapeutics Initiates Phase II Scleroderma Trial**
  Source: Reuters Medical News
  Date: June 24, 1996
  http://www.reuters.gov/archive/1996/06/24/professional/links/19960
  624xxxx005.html

- **Scleroderma Symptoms Develop In Three Patients Treated With Docetaxel**
  Source: Reuters Medical News
  Date: July 04, 1995
  http://www.reuters.gov/archive/1995/07/04/professional/links/19950
  704clin002.html

The NIH

Within MEDLINEplus, the NIH has made an agreement with the New York Times Syndicate, the AP News Service, and Reuters to deliver news that can be browsed by the public. Search news releases at **http://www.nlm.nih.gov/medlineplus/alphanews_a.html**. MEDLINEplus allows you to browse across an alphabetical index. Or you can search by date at **http://www.nlm.nih.gov/medlineplus/newsbydate.html**. Often, news items are indexed by MEDLINEplus within their search engine.

Business Wire

Business Wire is similar to PR Newswire. To access this archive, simply go to **http://www.businesswire.com**. You can scan the news by industry category or company name.

Internet Wire

Internet Wire is more focused on technology than the other wires. To access this site, go to **http://www.internetwire.com** and use the "Search Archive" option. Type in "scleroderma" (or synonyms). As this service is oriented to technology, you may wish to search for press releases covering diagnostic procedures or tests that you may have read about.

Search Engines

Free-to-view news can also be found in the news section of your favorite search engines (see the health news page at Yahoo: **http://dir.yahoo.com/Health/News_and_Media/,** or use this Web site's general news search page **http://news.yahoo.com/.** Type in "scleroderma" (or synonyms). If you know the name of a company that is relevant to scleroderma, you can go to any stock trading Web site (such as **www.etrade.com**) and search for the company name there. News items across various news sources are reported on indicated hyperlinks.

BBC

Covering news from a more European perspective, the British Broadcasting Corporation (BBC) allows the public free access to their news archive located at **http://www.bbc.co.uk/.** Search by "scleroderma" (or synonyms).

Newsletters on Scleroderma

Given their focus on current and relevant developments, newsletters are often more useful to patients than academic articles. You can find newsletters using the Combined Health Information Database (CHID). You will need to use the "Detailed Search" option. To access CHID, go directly to the following hyperlink: **http://chid.nih.gov/detail/detail.html**. Your investigation must limit the search to "Newsletter" and "scleroderma." Go to the bottom of the search page where "You may refine your search by." Select the dates and language that you prefer. For the format option, select "Newsletter." By making these selections and typing in "scleroderma" or synonyms into the "For these words:" box, you will only receive results on newsletters. The following list was generated using the options described above:

- **Beacon**

  Source: Peabody, MA: Scleroderma Federation, Inc. 1995. [20 p. average].

  Contact: Available from Scleroderma Federation, Inc. Peabody Office Building, 1 Newbury Street, Peabody, MA 01960. (800) 422-1113 or (508) 535-6600; FAX (508) 535-6696. Price: Free with membership.

  Summary: This newsletter presents information about scleroderma and the activities of the Scleroderma Federation, Inc. A typical issue includes articles on medical and social aspects of scleroderma, organizational news and announcements, updates in research and treatment, and letters to the editor.

- **Scleroderma Research Foundation**

  Source: Santa Barbara, CA: Scleroderma Research Foundation. 1994. 8 p. (average).

  Contact: Available from Scleroderma Research Foundation. 2320 Bath Street, Suite 307, Santa Barbara, CA 93105. (800) 441-2873 or (805) 563-9133; FAX (805) 563-2402. Price: Free with membership.

  Summary: This newsletter is intended for members of the Scleroderma Research Foundation. A typical issue includes articles on the medical and social aspects of scleroderma, news and announcements from the foundation, and information about current research activities.

Newsletter Articles

If you choose not to subscribe to a newsletter, you can nevertheless find references to newsletter articles. We recommend that you use the Combined Health Information Database, while limiting your search criteria to "newsletter articles." Again, you will need to use the "Detailed Search" option. Go to the following hyperlink: **http://chid.nih.gov/detail/detail.html**. Go to the bottom of the search page where "You may refine your search by." Select the dates and language that you prefer. For the format option, select "Newsletter Article."

By making these selections, and typing in "scleroderma" (or synonyms) into the "For these words:" box, you will only receive results on newsletter articles. You should check back periodically with this database as it is updated every 3 months. The following is a typical result when searching for newsletter articles on scleroderma:

- **Practical Tips for Living With Scleroderma**

  Source: Scleroderma Voice. p. 21-22. Winter 2000-2001.

  Contact: Available from Scleroderma Foundation. 12 Kent Way, Suite 101, Byfield, MA 01922. (800) 722-HOPE or (978) 463-5843. Fax (978) 463-5809. E-mail: sfinfo@scleroderma.org. Website: www.scleroderma.org.

  Summary: This newsletter article provides people who have scleroderma with information on practical tips for living with the disease. The article offers suggestions for grasping items with the fingers, coping with problems associated with eating and drinking, sitting comfortably, keeping the hands warm, bathing, sleeping, and dressing. General advice includes avoiding loose rugs or mats that can slip and cause falls and placing keys in a special attachment that can provide a better grip for holding and turning.

- **Update on Management of Scleroderma**

  Source: Bulletin on the Rheumatic Diseases. 49(10): 1-4. 2001.

  Contact: Available from Arthritis Foundation. 1330 West Peachtree Street, Atlanta, GA 30309. (404) 872-7100. Fax (404) 872-9559.

  Summary: This newsletter article provides health professionals with information on the management of scleroderma. This chronic disease targets the skin, heart, lungs, gastrointestinal tract, kidneys, muscles, and joints. Scleroderma is classified into limited and diffuse cutaneous forms. Almost all patients with scleroderma have Raynaud's phenomenon (RP). The most effective way to prevent RP is to avoid exposure to cold. Calcium channel blockers are currently the most effective and safest vasodilators for scleroderma related RP. Other useful medications include coated aspirin and intravenous prostaglandins. Options for managing gastrointestinal disease include elevating the head of the bed, using antacids, making dietary changes, and taking oral motility agents. Prostaglandins and their analogs are now available to treat pulmonary hypertension. Immunosuppressive agents can be useful in treating interstitial lung disease. Renal disease can be treated with angiotensin converting enzyme inhibitors. Disease modifying agents that can be used to treat early diffuse scleroderma include colchicine, paraaminobenzoic acid, and D-penicillamine. Other drugs that have been investigated for treating early diffuse scleroderma include relaxin, halofuginone, glucocorticoids, methotrexate, thalidomide, and cyclophosphamide. People who have scleroderma are more likely to experience major depression, so good pain control and the use of antidepressants are important. 1 table and 12 references.

- **Scleroderma and Dental Health**

  Source: Scleroderma Foundation Newsline. 2(3): 14-15. Summer-Fall 1999.

  Contact: Available from Scleroderma Foundation. 12 Kent Way, Suite 101, Byfield, MA 01922. (800) 722-4673 or (978) 463-5843. Fax (978) 463-5809. E-mail: sfinfo@scleroderma.org. Website: www.scleroderma.org.

  Summary: This newsletter article provides people who have scleroderma with information on oral and dental health. Common dental problems complicated by scleroderma include dental decay, periodontal disease, and loss of chewing ability. Tooth decay results from acid, which dissolves the hard outer coating of the tooth, creating a cavity in the dentin. Reducing dental decay involves eliminating decay producing bacteria from every tooth surface and applying fluoride to the teeth to make the enamel less easily dissolved by acid. Periodontal disease is also a concern for people who have scleroderma. One periodontal problem involves active infection of the tissue by harmful bacteria. Another results from the gradual tightening of the lips, cheeks, and gum tissues. As elasticity of these tissues is lost, a tough band of fibrous tissue connecting the inside of the lip to the gum tissue near the necks of the teeth can form. The article provides guidelines on selecting a toothbrush, removing plaque, and making dental visits easier. In addition, the article includes a list of products that people who have scleroderma may find helpful in treating their dental problems.

- **Laboratory Testing in Scleroderma**

  Source: Scleroderma Foundation Newsline. 2(3): 2,16-17,27. Summer-Fall 1999.

  Contact: Available from Scleroderma Foundation. 12 Kent Way, Suite 101, Byfield, MA 01922. (800) 722-4673 or (978) 463-5843. Fax (978) 463-5809. E-mail: sfinfo@scleroderma.org. Website: www.scleroderma.org.

  Summary: This newsletter article provides people who have scleroderma with information on the role of laboratory testing in diagnosing and following its course. Laboratory tests used to evaluate the status of scleroderma include those that assess blood count, hemoglobin and hematocrit, muscle enzymes, creatinine, blood urea nitrogen, urine tests, bilirubin, and alkaline phosphatase 5' nucleotidase. People who have scleroderma often have unique antibodies in their blood that can react with normal cell components. These antibodies are known as antinuclear antibodies (ANA). The ANA test is commonly used to assist in the diagnosis of scleroderma. Some autoantibodies have prognostic significance because they tend to be associated with milder or more severe forms of scleroderma. For example, antibodies to centromere proteins are associated with a limited form of scleroderma, but antibodies to topoisomerase 1 usually occur in people who have more widespread skin disease. Although certain autoantibodies have predictive value, ANA tests do have limitations. First, there is no correlation between the amount of autoantibodies in a given volume of blood and disease severity. Second, some patients occasionally change their antibodies completely. Third, scleroderma patients typically have more than one autoantibody. Research has attempted to determine whether autoantibodies hold clues to the etiology of scleroderma, but further research is still needed. 2 tables.

- **Scleroderma and Sexuality**

Source: The Beacon. 5(1):1,3,15,19-21; Winter 1997.

Contact: Available from Scleroderma Foundation. 12 Kent Way, Suite 101, Byfield, MA 01922. (800) 722-4673 or (978) 463-5843. Fax (978) 463-5809. E-mail: sfinfo@scleroderma.org. Website: www.scleroderma.org.

Summary: This newsletter article for health professionals and individuals with scleroderma presents available medical information on the effect of scleroderma symptoms on sexuality. Symptoms of scleroderma that can potentially affect sexuality are discussed, focusing on skin changes; calcinosis; joint pain and stiffness; muscle weakness; fixation of the fingers in a bent position; esophageal dysfunction; Raynaud's phenomenon; and lung, cardiac, and renal abnormalities. Specific problems for both women and men are highlighted. Suggestions for alleviating the negative effects of scleroderma on sexuality are offered, including altering the physical environment to enhance comfort during sexual activity, improving communication between sexual partners, making adjustments to accommodate hand deformities, and re-evaluating medications. In addition, the article highlights the intimate relationship problems confronting individuals with scleroderma and stresses the need for sexuality educators and therapists to help individuals with scleroderma improve the sexual aspect of their life.

- **Update on Scleroderma Kidney**

Source: The Beacon. 5(4):1,8-9. Fall 1997.

Contact: Available from Scleroderma Foundation. 12 Kent Way, Suite 101, Byfield, MA 01922. (800) 722-4673 or (978) 463-5843. Fax (978) 463-5809. E-mail: sfinfo@scleroderma.org. Website: www.scleroderma.org.

Summary: This newsletter article for individuals with scleroderma presents updated information on scleroderma kidney. It reviews the function of the normal kidney, explains the consequences of kidney failure, and describes the impact of scleroderma on kidney function. Although scleroderma kidney was the worst complication of scleroderma 25 years ago, significant advances in treatment have occurred, including the development of new blood pressure medications and the use of dialysis and transplantation. Despite these advances, researchers need to find a medication that will control blood pressure, allow healing of the lining of the blood vessels of the kidney, and reverse the blood flow problems within the kidney. 2 figures.

- **Spotlight On Scleroderma**

  Source: The Beacon. 4(2):14. Spring 1996.

  Contact: Available from Scleroderma Foundation. 12 Kent Way, Suite 101, Byfield, MA 01922. (800) 722-4673 or (978) 463-5843. Fax (978) 463-5809. E-mail: sfinfo@scleroderma.org. Website: www.scleroderma.org.

  Summary: This newsletter article for individuals with scleroderma reviews research on the role of mast cells in promoting inflammation in the skin in scleroderma patients. Mast cells appear in excess numbers in the skin around regions of scarring in scleroderma patients. Research shows that chemicals released from the mast cells signal fibroblasts to become activated. These fibroblasts then have the ability to cause immune cells to adhere to the fibroblast surface. Research also indicates that, in a skin-equivalent model system that mimics normal skin, fibroblasts express sticky molecules on their surface. These molecules capture white blood cells and cause them to stimulate attached fibroblasts, which probably leads to enhanced collagen production.

- **Living With Scleroderma Symptoms. A Personal Story: Part 5**

  Source: The Beacon. 4(2):6-7,15. Spring 1996.

  Contact: Available from Scleroderma Foundation. 12 Kent Way, Suite 101, Byfield, MA 01922. (800) 722-4673 or (978) 463-5843. Fax (978) 463-5809. E-mail: sfinfo@scleroderma.org. Website: www.scleroderma.org.

  Summary: This newsletter article for individuals with scleroderma presents the fifth part of a personal account of living with scleroderma symptoms. The gastrointestinal, pulmonary, and cutaneous manifestations of scleroderma that affected the author are discussed. He was affected by eating problems, such as food getting stuck part of the way down his esophagus; shortness of breathe and coughing when talking; and facial changes as a result of tightening of skin on his face. The way in which he has handled these symptoms is presented. 1 photograph.

- **Scleroderma and the Environment**

  Source: The Beacon. 4(2):1,5. Spring 1996.

  Contact: Available from Scleroderma Foundation. 12 Kent Way, Suite 101, Byfield, MA 01922. (800) 722-4673 or (978) 463-5843. Fax (978) 463-5809. E-mail: sfinfo@scleroderma.org. Website: www.scleroderma.org.

  Summary: This newsletter article for individuals with scleroderma identifies the environmental agents that have been implicated in scleroderma and pseudoscleroderma . The earliest environmental agent to be implicated as a cause of scleroderma was silica dust. Many studies have confirmed a relationship between silica exposure and diffuse cutaneous scleroderma . The association between silicone exposure and scleroderma is less clear because case-control studies have not found a real association but case reports have suggested a link between silicone exposure and scleroderma . Examples of pseudoscleroderma occurring after ingestion of chemicals or drugs are the toxic oil syndrome epidemic that occurred in Spain in 1981 and the contaminated L-tryptophan epidemic that occurred mainly in the United States in 1989. In addition, exposure to vinyl chloride monomer; organic solvents; and drugs such as bleomycin , pentazocine , and various appetite suppressants have been associated with scleroderma or pseudoscleroderma .

- **Natural History and Treatment of Scleroderma**

  Source: The Beacon. 3(4):1,13-17; Fall 1995.

  Contact: Scleroderma Federation, Peabody, MA 01940.

  Summary: This newsletter article for health professionals, the first of a two-part series, focuses on the natural history and treatment of scleroderma. The use of skin scoring to assess overall skin thickness is described. The characteristics of the skin in limited and diffuse cutaneous scleroderma are presented. The complications that individuals with these forms of scleroderma may develop are highlighted. Lung disease in individuals with scleroderma is discussed. Suggestions for the non pharmacological management of Raynaud's phenomenon are presented. Pharmacologic agents considered effective in treating Raynaud's phenomenon are listed. Suggestions for conducting effective studies on medications used to treat Raynaud's phenomenon are provided. Questions and answers about scleroderma are also presented.

- **Scleroderma: It Can Damage Skin and Much More**

  Source: Mayo Clinic Health Letter. 18(10): 6. October 2000.

  Contact: Available from Mayo Clinic Health Letter, 200 First Street SW, Rochester, MN 55905. (800) 333-9037 or (303) 604-1465. Email: HealthLetter@Mayo.edu.

  Summary: This newsletter article provides people who have scleroderma with information on this progressive disease, which leads to a hardening and scarring of the skin and connective tissues. Scleroderma results from the overproduction and accumulation of collagen in body tissues. Types of scleroderma include morphea and systemic progressive sclerosis. The former is a localized type of scleroderma that usually affects the hands, face, arms, or legs. The latter often involves internal organs as well as the skin. Laboratory tests might be needed to diagnose the disease. There is no cure for scleroderma, so it is usually managed by treating the symptoms. Treatment options include skin protection measures, drug therapy, and exercise.

- **Medical Briefs: Childhood Localized Scleroderma**

  Source: Scleroderma Foundation Newsletter. 1(2): 1,10-11. Spring 1998.

  Contact: Available from Scleroderma Foundation. 12 Kent Way, Suite 101, Byfield, MA 01922. (800) 722-4673 or (978) 463-5843. Fax (978) 463-5809. E-mail: sfinfo@scleroderma.org. Website: www.scleroderma.org.

  Summary: This newsletter article provides health professionals with information on the clinical presentation, etiology, diagnosis, prognosis, and treatment of morphea and linear scleroderma in children. These two types of the localized form are closely related to juvenile arthritis, and they can occur in the same patient. Morphea can occur either as a single plaque or as a small group of plaques, which can be small or large. Different forms of morphea produce different patterns of plaques, while linear scleroderma forms plaques in long streaks or bands that may extend the length of the arm or leg. Theories about the etiology of morphea and linear scleroderma involve vascular damage and autoimmunity. There is no definitive laboratory test to diagnose these disorders. Microscopic analysis of the nailfolds of the fingers is a noninvasive diagnostic method. Prognosis depends on the extent of skin involvement, functional impairment, and any complications that may develop. Treatment options are directed at relieving symptoms, since there is no cure for these conditions. Strategies that may increase patient comfort include maintaining good skin care; protecting the body from cold; using heat, massage, or physical therapy; exercising; and using anti-inflammatory drugs to relieve associated muscle and joint pain.

- **Therapy-Treatment of Systemic Sclerosis**

  Source: Scleroderma Voice. p. 12-14. Winter 2000-2001.

  Contact: Available from Scleroderma Foundation. 12 Kent Way, Suite 101, Byfield, MA 01922. (800) 722-HOPE or (978) 463-5843. Fax (978) 463-5809. E-mail: sfinfo@scleroderma.org. Website: www.scleroderma.org.

  Summary: This newsletter article provides health professionals and people who have scleroderma with information on approaches to treating systemic sclerosis (SSc). Interrupting the pathogenetic cycle is a reasonable approach to the treatment of SSc. Treatment might be aimed at addressing the vascular damage, preventing fibrosis, or suppressing the immune response. The article highlights the results of recent clinical trials of a prostacyclin derivative, iloprost, interferon gamma, D-penicillamine, chlorambucil, cyclosporine A, methotrexate, and cyclophosphamide. In general, these trials support the use of prostacyclin derivatives, antifibrotic regimens, and immunosuppressive agents to treat SSc. A more definitive test of the usefulness of immunosuppression for SSc is a trial of stem cell transplantation (SCT). Although SCT results have been encouraging, there has been almost a 25 percent mortality rate among SCT treated patients.

- **Less Well-Recognized Manifestations of Systemic Sclerosis (Scleroderma)**

  Source: Scleroderma Foundation Newsline. 2(3): 3,26-27. Summer-Fall 1999.

  Contact: Available from Scleroderma Foundation. 12 Kent Way, Suite 101, Byfield, MA 01922. (800) 722-4673 or (978) 463-5843. Fax (978) 463-5809. E-mail: sfinfo@scleroderma.org. Website: www.scleroderma.org.

  Summary: This newsletter article provides people who have scleroderma with the less well recognized manifestations of systemic sclerosis. Skin induration and fibrosis, as well as the manifestations of the CREST syndrome, are well known clinical manifestations of systemic sclerosis. However, there are several other clinical manifestations that are not as well recognized, including hypothyroidism, impotence, bladder fibrosis, testicular fibrosis, carpal tunnel syndrome, trigeminal nerve palsy, periodontal ligament resorption, and vocal cord infiltration. Hypothyroidism manifests as progressive weight gain, decreased tolerance to cold temperatures, sluggishness, slowing of mental functions, and, in later stages, cutaneous lesions in the lower extremities. Thyroid hormone replacement often improves these manifestations. Impotence may be the result of generalized fatigue, the effect the disease has on the body, or psychological factors. However, it may be directly caused by the pathologic alterations of the disease. Various therapeutic measures are needed to successfully overcome the difficulties associated with this manifestation of systemic sclerosis. Bladder manifestations include an urgent need to urinate and increased frequency of urination. Various tests may be used to determine whether systemic sclerosis or other problems are responsible for symptoms. Testicular fibrosis manifests by enlargement of the testicles. Carpal tunnel syndrome is occasionally one of the earliest manifestations of systemic sclerosis. Trigeminal nerve palsy, which is less common than carpal tunnel syndrome, causes pain and loss of sensation in the lower part of the face on just one side. Periodontal ligament resorption may produce pain at the root of the affected teeth. Vocal cord involvement results in severe, persistent, and progressive hoarseness.

Academic Periodicals covering Scleroderma

Academic periodicals can be a highly technical yet valuable source of information on scleroderma. We have compiled the following list of periodicals known to publish articles relating to scleroderma and which are currently indexed within the National Library of Medicine's PubMed database (follow hyperlinks to view more information, summaries, etc., for each). In addition to these sources, to keep current on articles written on scleroderma published by any of the periodicals listed below, you can simply follow the hyperlink indicated or go to the following Web site: **www.ncbi.nlm.nih.gov/pubmed**. Type the periodical's name into the search box to find the latest studies published.

If you want complete details about the historical contents of a periodical, you can also visit **http://www.ncbi.nlm.nih.gov/entrez/jrbrowser.cgi**. Here, type in the name of the journal or its abbreviation, and you will receive an index of published articles. At **http://locatorplus.gov/** you can retrieve more indexing information on medical periodicals (e.g. the name of the publisher). Select the button "Search LOCATORplus." Then type in the name of the journal and select the advanced search option "Journal Title Search." The following is a sample of periodicals which publish articles on scleroderma:

- **Advances in Experimental Medicine and Biology. (Adv Exp Med Biol)**
  http://www.ncbi.nlm.nih.gov/entrez/jrbrowser.cgi?field=0&regexp=Advances+in+Experimental+Medicine+and+Biology&dispmax=20&dispstart=0

- **Annals of the New York Academy of Sciences. (Ann N Y Acad Sci)**
  http://www.ncbi.nlm.nih.gov/entrez/jrbrowser.cgi?field=0&regexp=Annals+of+the+New+York+Academy+of+Sciences&dispmax=20&dispstart=0

- **Annals of the Rheumatic Diseases. (Ann Rheum Dis)**
  http://www.ncbi.nlm.nih.gov/entrez/jrbrowser.cgi?field=0&regexp=Annals+of+the+Rheumatic+Diseases&dispmax=20&dispstart=0

- **Archives of Dermatology. (Arch Dermatol)**
  http://www.ncbi.nlm.nih.gov/entrez/jrbrowser.cgi?field=0&regexp=Archives+of+Dermatology&dispmax=20&dispstart=0

- **Archives of Physical Medicine and Rehabilitation. (Arch Phys Med Rehabil)**
  http://www.ncbi.nlm.nih.gov/entrez/jrbrowser.cgi?field=0&regexp=Archives+of+Physical+Medicine+and+Rehabilitation&dispmax=20&dispstart=0

- **Arthritis and Rheumatism. (Arthritis Rheum)**
  http://www.ncbi.nlm.nih.gov/entrez/jrbrowser.cgi?field=0&regexp=Arthritis+and+Rheumatism&dispmax=20&dispstart=0

- **Arthritis Research. (Arthritis Res)**
  http://www.ncbi.nlm.nih.gov/entrez/jrbrowser.cgi?field=0&regexp=Arthritis+Research&dispmax=20&dispstart=0

- **Journal of Behavioral Medicine. (J Behav Med)**
  http://www.ncbi.nlm.nih.gov/entrez/jrbrowser.cgi?field=0&regexp=Journal+of+Behavioral+Medicine&dispmax=20&dispstart=0

- **Journal of Dermatological Science. (J Dermatol Sci)**
  http://www.ncbi.nlm.nih.gov/entrez/jrbrowser.cgi?field=0&regexp=Journal+of+Dermatological+Science&dispmax=20&dispstart=0

- **Scandinavian Journal of Gastroenterology. (Scand J Gastroenterol)**
  http://www.ncbi.nlm.nih.gov/entrez/jrbrowser.cgi?field=0&regexp=Sc
  andinavian+Journal+of+Gastroenterology&dispmax=20&dispstart=0

- **Seminars in Arthritis and Rheumatism. (Semin Arthritis Rheum)**
  http://www.ncbi.nlm.nih.gov/entrez/jrbrowser.cgi?field=0&regexp=Se
  minars+in+Arthritis+and+Rheumatism&dispmax=20&dispstart=0

- **The Journal of Cell Biology. (J Cell Biol)**
  http://www.ncbi.nlm.nih.gov/entrez/jrbrowser.cgi?field=0&regexp=Th
  e+Journal+of+Cell+Biology&dispmax=20&dispstart=0

- **The Journal of Hand Surgery. (J Hand Surg [Am])**
  http://www.ncbi.nlm.nih.gov/entrez/jrbrowser.cgi?field=0&regexp=Th
  e+Journal+of+Hand+Surgery&dispmax=20&dispstart=0

- **The Journal of Investigative Dermatology. (J Invest Dermatol)**
  http://www.ncbi.nlm.nih.gov/entrez/jrbrowser.cgi?field=0&regexp=Th
  e+Journal+of+Investigative+Dermatology&dispmax=20&dispstart=0

- **The Journal of Pathology. (J Pathol)**
  http://www.ncbi.nlm.nih.gov/entrez/jrbrowser.cgi?field=0&regexp=Th
  e+Journal+of+Pathology&dispmax=20&dispstart=0

- **The Medical Journal of Australia. (Med J Aust)**
  http://www.ncbi.nlm.nih.gov/entrez/jrbrowser.cgi?field=0&regexp=Th
  e+Medical+Journal+of+Australia&dispmax=20&dispstart=0

Vocabulary Builder

Alkaline: Having the reactions of an alkali. [EU]

Antidepressant: An agent that stimulates the mood of a depressed patient, including tricyclic antidepressants and monoamine oxidase inhibitors. [EU]

Bilirubin: A bile pigment that is a degradation product of heme. [NIH]

Elasticity: Resistance and recovery from distortion of shape. [NIH]

Hematocrit: Measurement of the volume of packed red cells in a blood specimen by centrifugation. The procedure is performed using a tube with graduated markings or with automated blood cell counters. It is used as an indicator of erythrocyte status in disease. For example, anemia shows a low hematocrit, polycythemia, high values. [NIH]

Hoarseness: An unnaturally deep or rough quality of voice. [NIH]

Hypothyroidism: Deficiency of thyroid activity. In adults, it is most common in women and is characterized by decrease in basal metabolic rate, tiredness and lethargy, sensitivity to cold, and menstrual disturbances. If untreated, it progresses to full-blown myxoedema. In infants, severe hypothyroidism leads to cretinism. In juveniles, the manifestations are intermediate, with less severe mental and developmental retardation and only mild symptoms of the adult form. When due to pituitary deficiency of thyrotropin secretion it is called secondary hypothyroidism. [EU]

Impotence: The inability to perform sexual intercourse. [NIH]

Ingestion: The act of taking food, medicines, etc., into the body, by mouth. [EU]

Intravenous: Within a vein or veins. [EU]

Ligament: A band of fibrous tissue that connects bones or cartilages, serving to support and strengthen joints. [EU]

Nitrogen: An element with the atomic symbol N, atomic number 7, and atomic weight 14. Nitrogen exists as a diatomic gas and makes up about 78% of the earth's atmosphere by volume. It is a constituent of proteins and nucleic acids and found in all living cells. [NIH]

Perforation: 1. the act of boring or piercing through a part. 2. a hole made through a part or substance. [EU]

Resorption: The loss of substance through physiologic or pathologic means, such as loss of dentin and cementum of a tooth, or of the alveolar process of the mandible or maxilla. [EU]

Testicular: Pertaining to a testis. [EU]

Thyrotropin: A peptide hormone secreted by the anterior pituitary. It promotes the growth of the thyroid gland and stimulates the synthesis of thyroid hormones and the release of thyroxine by the thyroid gland. [NIH]

Tolerance: 1. the ability to endure unusually large doses of a drug or toxin. 2. acquired drug tolerance; a decreasing response to repeated constant doses of a drug or the need for increasing doses to maintain a constant response. [EU]

CHAPTER 9. PHYSICIAN GUIDELINES AND DATABASES

Overview

Doctors and medical researchers rely on a number of information sources to help patients with their conditions. Many will subscribe to journals or newsletters published by their professional associations or refer to specialized textbooks or clinical guides published for the medical profession. In this chapter, we focus on databases and Internet-based guidelines created or written for this professional audience.

NIH Guidelines

For the more common diseases, The National Institutes of Health publish guidelines that are frequently consulted by physicians. Publications are typically written by one or more of the various NIH Institutes. For physician guidelines, commonly referred to as "clinical" or "professional" guidelines, you can visit the following Institutes:

- Office of the Director (OD); guidelines consolidated across agencies available at **http://www.nih.gov/health/consumer/conkey.htm**

- National Institute of General Medical Sciences (NIGMS); fact sheets available at **http://www.nigms.nih.gov/news/facts/**

- National Library of Medicine (NLM); extensive encyclopedia (A.D.A.M., Inc.) with guidelines:
  http://www.nlm.nih.gov/medlineplus/healthtopics.html

- National Institute of Arthritis and Musculoskeletal and Skin Diseases (NIAMS); fact sheets and guidelines available at
  http://www.nih.gov/niams/healthinfo/

NIH Databases

In addition to the various Institutes of Health that publish professional guidelines, the NIH has designed a number of databases for professionals.[28] Physician-oriented resources provide a wide variety of information related to the biomedical and health sciences, both past and present. The format of these resources varies. Searchable databases, bibliographic citations, full text articles (when available), archival collections, and images are all available. The following are referenced by the National Library of Medicine:[29]

- **Bioethics:** Access to published literature on the ethical, legal and public policy issues surrounding healthcare and biomedical research. This information is provided in conjunction with the Kennedy Institute of Ethics located at Georgetown University, Washington, D.C.: **http://www.nlm.nih.gov/databases/databases_bioethics.html**

- **HIV/AIDS Resources:** Describes various links and databases dedicated to HIV/AIDS research: **http://www.nlm.nih.gov/pubs/factsheets/aidsinfs.html**

- **NLM Online Exhibitions:** Describes "Exhibitions in the History of Medicine": **http://www.nlm.nih.gov/exhibition/exhibition.html**. Additional resources for historical scholarship in medicine: **http://www.nlm.nih.gov/hmd/hmd.html**

- **Biotechnology Information:** Access to public databases. The National Center for Biotechnology Information conducts research in computational biology, develops software tools for analyzing genome data, and disseminates biomedical information for the better understanding of molecular processes affecting human health and disease: **http://www.ncbi.nlm.nih.gov/**

- **Population Information:** The National Library of Medicine provides access to worldwide coverage of population, family planning, and related health issues, including family planning technology and programs, fertility, and population law and policy: **http://www.nlm.nih.gov/databases/databases_population.html**

- **Cancer Information:** Access to caner-oriented databases: **http://www.nlm.nih.gov/databases/databases_cancer.html**

---

[28] Remember, for the general public, the National Library of Medicine recommends the databases referenced in MEDLINE*plus* (**http://medlineplus.gov/** or **http://www.nlm.nih.gov/medlineplus/databases.html**).

[29] See http://www.nlm.nih.gov/databases/databases.html.

- **Profiles in Science:** Offering the archival collections of prominent twentieth-century biomedical scientists to the public through modern digital technology: **http://www.profiles.nlm.nih.gov/**

- **Chemical Information:** Provides links to various chemical databases and references: **http://sis.nlm.nih.gov/Chem/ChemMain.html**

- **Clinical Alerts:** Reports the release of findings from the NIH-funded clinical trials where such release could significantly affect morbidity and mortality: **http://www.nlm.nih.gov/databases/alerts/clinical_alerts.html**

- **Space Life Sciences:** Provides links and information to space-based research (including NASA): **http://www.nlm.nih.gov/databases/databases_space.html**

- **MEDLINE:** Bibliographic database covering the fields of medicine, nursing, dentistry, veterinary medicine, the healthcare system, and the pre-clinical sciences: **http://www.nlm.nih.gov/databases/databases_medline.html**

- **Toxicology and Environmental Health Information (TOXNET):** Databases covering toxicology and environmental health: **http://sis.nlm.nih.gov/Tox/ToxMain.html**

- **Visible Human Interface:** Anatomically detailed, three-dimensional representations of normal male and female human bodies: **http://www.nlm.nih.gov/research/visible/visible_human.html**

While all of the above references may be of interest to physicians who study and treat scleroderma, the following are particularly noteworthy.

The Combined Health Information Database

A comprehensive source of information on clinical guidelines written for professionals is the Combined Health Information Database. You will need to limit your search to "Brochure/Pamphlet," "Fact Sheet," or "Information Package" and scleroderma using the "Detailed Search" option. Go directly to the following hyperlink: **http://chid.nih.gov/detail/detail.html**. To find associations, use the drop boxes at the bottom of the search page where "You may refine your search by." For the publication date, select "All Years," select your preferred language, and the format option "Fact Sheet." By making these selections and typing "scleroderma" (or synonyms) into the "For these words:" box above, you will only receive results on fact sheets dealing with scleroderma. The following is a sample result:

- **Sexuality in Scleroderma**

  Source: Watsonville, CA: United Scleroderma Foundation Inc. 1990. 4 p.

  Contact: Available from United Scleroderma Foundation Inc. P.O. Box 350, Watsonville, CA 95077. (408) 728-2202. Price: $0.20.

  Summary: The United Scleroderma Foundation has published a number of brochures intended to give scleroderma patients a better understanding of their illness and to extend encouragement in coping with the difficulties of daily living. This brochure was produced in an effort to aid patients in dealing with scleroderma and sexuality. The authors note that scleroderma is a chronic disease, difficult to diagnose, and requiring understanding, communication, and support as vital factors in patients coping with the disease. Topics include self image; the role of health professionals; sexual functioning and scleroderma; physical concerns related to women; contraception; pregnancy; physical concerns related to men; using condoms; renal problems; Peyronie's disease; and resources for additional help. The addresses of five resource organizations conclude the brochure.

- **Understanding and Managing Scleroderma**

  Source: Peabody, MA: Scleroderma Federation, Inc. March 1994. 36 p.

  Contact: Available from Scleroderma Federation, Inc. Peabody Office Building, 1 Newbury Street, Peabody, MA 01960. (800) 422-1113 or (508) 535-6600; FAX (508) 535-6696. Price: Free.

  Summary: This booklet is written for persons with scleroderma and their families. Information is presented about the characteristics and symptoms of scleroderma, diagnosis, and treatment of symptoms. The booklet also offers suggestions to patients about what they can do to help themselves and their physicians in the management of the disease and answers several frequently asked questions about scleroderma.

- **About Scleroderma**

  Source: Peabody, MA: Scleroderma Federation, Inc. [6 p.].

  Contact: Available from Scleroderma Federation, Inc. Peabody Office Building, 1 Newbury Street, Peabody, MA 01960. (800) 422-1113 or (508) 535-6600; FAX (508) 535-6696. Price: Free.

  Summary: This brochure presents general information about scleroderma, a chronic and progressive illness caused by an overproduction of collagen. Symptoms of scleroderma, diagnosis, treatments, and suggestions for self-care are described. Drug therapy research is also briefly discussed.

The NLM Gateway[30]

The NLM (National Library of Medicine) Gateway is a Web-based system that lets users search simultaneously in multiple retrieval systems at the U.S. National Library of Medicine (NLM). It allows users of NLM services to initiate searches from one Web interface, providing "one-stop searching" for many of NLM's information resources or databases.[31] One target audience for the Gateway is the Internet user who is new to NLM's online resources and does not know what information is available or how best to search for it. This audience may include physicians and other healthcare providers, researchers, librarians, students, and, increasingly, patients, their families, and the public.[32] To use the NLM Gateway, simply go to the search site at **http://gateway.nlm.nih.gov/gw/Cmd**. Type "scleroderma" (or synonyms) into the search box and click "Search." The results will be presented in a tabular form, indicating the number of references in each database category.

Results Summary

Category	Items Found
Journal Articles	345501
Books / Periodicals / Audio Visual	2567
Consumer Health	294
Meeting Abstracts	3093
Other Collections	100
Total	351555

---

[30] Adapted from NLM: **http://gateway.nlm.nih.gov/gw/Cmd?Overview.x**.

[31] The NLM Gateway is currently being developed by the Lister Hill National Center for Biomedical Communications (LHNCBC) at the National Library of Medicine (NLM) of the National Institutes of Health (NIH).

[32] Other users may find the Gateway useful for an overall search of NLM's information resources. Some searchers may locate what they need immediately, while others will utilize the Gateway as an adjunct tool to other NLM search services such as PubMed® and MEDLINEplus®. The Gateway connects users with multiple NLM retrieval systems while also providing a search interface for its own collections. These collections include various types of information that do not logically belong in PubMed, LOCATORplus, or other established NLM retrieval systems (e.g., meeting announcements and pre-1966 journal citations). The Gateway will provide access to the information found in an increasing number of NLM retrieval systems in several phases.

HSTAT[33]

HSTAT is a free, Web-based resource that provides access to full-text documents used in healthcare decision-making.[34] HSTAT's audience includes healthcare providers, health service researchers, policy makers, insurance companies, consumers, and the information professionals who serve these groups. HSTAT provides access to a wide variety of publications, including clinical practice guidelines, quick-reference guides for clinicians, consumer health brochures, evidence reports and technology assessments from the Agency for Healthcare Research and Quality (AHRQ), as well as AHRQ's Put Prevention Into Practice.[35] Simply search by "scleroderma" (or synonyms) at the following Web site: **http://text.nlm.nih.gov**.

Coffee Break: Tutorials for Biologists[36]

Some patients may wish to have access to a general healthcare site that takes a scientific view of the news and covers recent breakthroughs in biology that may one day assist physicians in developing treatments. To this end, we recommend "Coffee Break," a collection of short reports on recent biological discoveries. Each report incorporates interactive tutorials that demonstrate how bioinformatics tools are used as a part of the research process. Currently, all Coffee Breaks are written by NCBI staff.[37] Each report is about 400 words and is usually based on a discovery reported in one or more articles from recently published, peer-reviewed literature.[38] This site has new

---

[33] Adapted from HSTAT: http://www.nlm.nih.gov/pubs/factsheets/hstat.html.

[34] The HSTAT URL is **http://hstat.nlm.nih.gov/**.

[35] Other important documents in HSTAT include: the National Institutes of Health (NIH) Consensus Conference Reports and Technology Assessment Reports; the HIV/AIDS Treatment Information Service (ATIS) resource documents; the Substance Abuse and Mental Health Services Administration's Center for Substance Abuse Treatment (SAMHSA/CSAT) Treatment Improvement Protocols (TIP) and Center for Substance Abuse Prevention (SAMHSA/CSAP) Prevention Enhancement Protocols System (PEPS); the Public Health Service (PHS) Preventive Services Task Force's *Guide to Clinical Preventive Services*; the independent, nonfederal Task Force on Community Services *Guide to Community Preventive Services*; and the Health Technology Advisory Committee (HTAC) of the Minnesota Health Care Commission (MHCC) health technology evaluations.

[36] Adapted from http://www.ncbi.nlm.nih.gov/Coffeebreak/Archive/FAQ.html.

[37] The figure that accompanies each article is frequently supplied by an expert external to NCBI, in which case the source of the figure is cited. The result is an interactive tutorial that tells a biological story.

[38] After a brief introduction that sets the work described into a broader context, the report focuses on how a molecular understanding can provide explanations of observed biology and lead to therapies for diseases. Each vignette is accompanied by a figure and hypertext links that lead to a series of pages that interactively show how NCBI tools and resources are used in the research process.

articles every few weeks, so it can be considered an online magazine of sorts, and intended for general background information. You can access the Coffee Break Web site at **http://www.ncbi.nlm.nih.gov/Coffeebreak/**.

Other Commercial Databases

In addition to resources maintained by official agencies, other databases exist that are commercial ventures addressing medical professionals. Here are a few examples that may interest you:

- **CliniWeb International:** Index and table of contents to selected clinical information on the Internet; see **http://www.ohsu.edu/cliniweb/**.

- **Image Engine:** Multimedia electronic medical record system that integrates a wide range of digitized clinical images with textual data stored in the University of Pittsburgh Medical Center's MARS electronic medical record system; see the following Web site: **http://www.cml.upmc.edu/cml/imageengine/imageEngine.html**.

- **Medical World Search:** Searches full text from thousands of selected medical sites on the Internet; see **http://www.mwsearch.com/**.

- **MedWeaver:** Prototype system that allows users to search differential diagnoses for any list of signs and symptoms, to search medical literature, and to explore relevant Web sites; see **http://www.med.virginia.edu/~wmd4n/medweaver.html**.

- **Metaphrase:** Middleware component intended for use by both caregivers and medical records personnel. It converts the informal language generally used by caregivers into terms from formal, controlled vocabularies; see the following Web site: **http://www.lexical.com/Metaphrase.html**.

The Genome Project and Scleroderma

With all the discussion in the press about the Human Genome Project, it is only natural that physicians, researchers, and patients want to know about how human genes relate to scleroderma. In the following section, we will discuss databases and references used by physicians and scientists who work in this area.

Online Mendelian Inheritance in Man (OMIM)

The Online Mendelian Inheritance in Man (OMIM) database is a catalog of human genes and genetic disorders authored and edited by Dr. Victor A. McKusick and his colleagues at Johns Hopkins and elsewhere. OMIM was developed for the World Wide Web by the National Center for Biotechnology Information (NCBI).[39] The database contains textual information, pictures, and reference information. It also contains copious links to NCBI's Entrez database of MEDLINE articles and sequence information.

Go to **http://www.ncbi.nlm.nih.gov/Omim/searchomim.html** to search the database. Type "scleroderma" (or synonyms) in the search box, and click "Submit Search." If too many results appear, you can narrow the search by adding the word "clinical." Each report will have additional links to related research and databases. By following these links, especially the link titled "Database Links," you will be exposed to numerous specialized databases that are largely used by the scientific community. These databases are overly technical and seldom used by the general public, but offer an abundance of information. The following is an example of the results you can obtain from the OMIM for scleroderma:

- **Polymyositis/scleroderma Autoantigen 1**
  Web site: http://www.ncbi.nlm.nih.gov/htbin-post/Omim/dispmim?606180

- **Polymyositis/scleroderma Autoantigen 2**
  Web site: http://www.ncbi.nlm.nih.gov/htbin-post/Omim/dispmim?605960

- **Scleroderma, Familial Progressive**
  Web site: http://www.ncbi.nlm.nih.gov/htbin-post/Omim/dispmim?181750

- **Sjogren Syndrome/scleroderma Autoantigen 1**
  Web site: http://www.ncbi.nlm.nih.gov/htbin-post/Omim/dispmim?606044

---

[39] Adapted from **http://www.ncbi.nlm.nih.gov/**. Established in 1988 as a national resource for molecular biology information, NCBI creates public databases, conducts research in computational biology, develops software tools for analyzing genome data, and disseminates biomedical information--all for the better understanding of molecular processes affecting human health and disease.

Genes and Disease (NCBI - Map)

The Genes and Disease database is produced by the National Center for Biotechnology Information of the National Library of Medicine at the National Institutes of Health. This Web site categorizes each disorder by the system of the body associated with it. Go to **http://www.ncbi.nlm.nih.gov/disease/**, and browse the system pages to have a full view of important conditions linked to human genes. Since this site is regularly updated, you may wish to re-visit it from time to time. The following systems and associated disorders are addressed:

- **Cancer:** Uncontrolled cell division.
  Examples: Breast And Ovarian Cancer, Burkitt lymphoma, chronic myeloid leukemia, colon cancer, lung cancer, malignant melanoma, multiple endocrine neoplasia, neurofibromatosis, p53 tumor suppressor, pancreatic cancer, prostate cancer, Ras oncogene, RB: retinoblastoma, von Hippel-Lindau syndrome.
  Web site: **http://www.ncbi.nlm.nih.gov/disease/Cancer.html**

- **Immune System:** Fights invaders.
  Examples: Asthma, autoimmune polyglandular syndrome, Crohn's disease, DiGeorge syndrome, familial Mediterranean fever, immunodeficiency with Hyper-IgM, severe combined immunodeficiency.
  Web site: **http://www.ncbi.nlm.nih.gov/disease/Immune.html**

- **Metabolism:** Food and energy.
  Examples: Adreno-leukodystrophy, Atherosclerosis, Best disease, Gaucher disease, Glucose galactose malabsorption, Gyrate atrophy, Juvenile onset diabetes, Obesity, Paroxysmal nocturnal hemoglobinuria, Phenylketonuria, Refsum disease, Tangier disease, Tay-Sachs disease.
  Web site: **http://www.ncbi.nlm.nih.gov/disease/Mctabolism.html**

- **Muscle and Bone:** Movement and growth.
  Examples: Duchenne muscular dystrophy, Ellis-van Creveld syndrome, Marfan syndrome, myotonic dystrophy, spinal muscular atrophy.
  Web site: **http://www.ncbi.nlm.nih.gov/disease/Muscle.html**

- **Nervous System:** Mind and body.
  Examples: Alzheimer disease, Amyotrophic lateral sclerosis, Angelman syndrome, Charcot-Marie-Tooth disease, epilepsy, essential tremor, Fragile X syndrome, Friedreich's ataxia, Huntington disease, Niemann-Pick disease, Parkinson disease, Prader-Willi syndrome, Rett syndrome, Spinocerebellar atrophy, Williams syndrome.
  Web site: **http://www.ncbi.nlm.nih.gov/disease/Brain.html**

- **Signals:** Cellular messages.
  Examples: Ataxia telangiectasia, Baldness, Cockayne syndrome, Glaucoma, SRY: sex determination, Tuberous sclerosis, Waardenburg syndrome, Werner syndrome.
  Web site: **http://www.ncbi.nlm.nih.gov/disease/Signals.html**

- **Transporters:** Pumps and channels.
  Examples: Cystic Fibrosis, deafness, diastrophic dysplasia, Hemophilia A, long-QT syndrome, Menkes syndrome, Pendred syndrome, polycystic kidney disease, sickle cell anemia, Wilson's disease, Zellweger syndrome.
  Web site: **http://www.ncbi.nlm.nih.gov/disease/Transporters.html**

Entrez

Entrez is a search and retrieval system that integrates several linked databases at the National Center for Biotechnology Information (NCBI). These databases include nucleotide sequences, protein sequences, macromolecular structures, whole genomes, and MEDLINE through PubMed. Entrez provides access to the following databases:

- **PubMed:** Biomedical literature (PubMed),
  Web site: **http://www.ncbi.nlm.nih.gov/entrez/query.fcgi?db=PubMed**

- **Nucleotide Sequence Database (Genbank):**
  Web site:
  http://www.ncbi.nlm.nih.gov/entrez/query.fcgi?db=Nucleotide

- **Protein Sequence Database:**
  Web site: **http://www.ncbi.nlm.nih.gov/entrez/query.fcgi?db=Protein**

- **Structure:** Three-dimensional macromolecular structures,
  Web site: **http://www.ncbi.nlm.nih.gov/entrez/query.fcgi?db=Structure**

- **Genome:** Complete genome assemblies,
  Web site: **http://www.ncbi.nlm.nih.gov/entrez/query.fcgi?db=Genome**

- **PopSet:** Population study data sets,
  Web site: **http://www.ncbi.nlm.nih.gov/entrez/query.fcgi?db=Popset**

- **OMIM:** Online Mendelian Inheritance in Man,
  Web site: **http://www.ncbi.nlm.nih.gov/entrez/query.fcgi?db=OMIM**

- **Taxonomy:** Organisms in GenBank,
  Web site:
  http://www.ncbi.nlm.nih.gov/entrez/query.fcgi?db=Taxonomy

- **Books:** Online books,
  Web site: **http://www.ncbi.nlm.nih.gov/entrez/query.fcgi?db=books**

- **ProbeSet:** Gene Expression Omnibus (GEO),
  Web site: **http://www.ncbi.nlm.nih.gov/entrez/query.fcgi?db=geo**

- **3D Domains:** Domains from Entrez Structure,
  Web site: **http://www.ncbi.nlm.nih.gov/entrez/query.fcgi?db=geo**

- **NCBI's Protein Sequence Information Survey Results:**
  Web site: **http://www.ncbi.nlm.nih.gov/About/proteinsurvey/**

To access the Entrez system at the National Center for Biotechnology Information, go to **http://www.ncbi.nlm.nih.gov/entrez/**, and then select the database that you would like to search. The databases available are listed in the drop box next to "Search." In the box next to "for," enter "scleroderma" (or synonyms) and click "Go."

Jablonski's Multiple Congenital Anomaly/Mental Retardation (MCA/MR) Syndromes Database[40]

This online resource can be quite useful. It has been developed to facilitate the identification and differentiation of syndromic entities. Special attention is given to the type of information that is usually limited or completely omitted in existing reference sources due to space limitations of the printed form.

At **http://www.nlm.nih.gov/mesh/jablonski/syndrome_toc/toc_a.html** you can also search across syndromes using an alphabetical index. You can also search at **http://www.nlm.nih.gov/mesh/jablonski/syndrome_db.html**.

The Genome Database[41]

Established at Johns Hopkins University in Baltimore, Maryland in 1990, the Genome Database (GDB) is the official central repository for genomic mapping data resulting from the Human Genome Initiative. In the spring of 1999, the Bioinformatics Supercomputing Centre (BiSC) at the Hospital for Sick Children in Toronto, Ontario assumed the management of GDB. The Human Genome Initiative is a worldwide research effort focusing on structural analysis of human DNA to determine the location and sequence of the estimated 100,000 human genes. In support of this project, GDB stores

---

[40] Adapted from the National Library of Medicine:
http://www.nlm.nih.gov/mesh/jablonski/about_syndrome.html.
[41] Adapted from the Genome Database:
http://gdbwww.gdb.org/gdb/aboutGDB.html#mission.

and curates data generated by researchers worldwide who are engaged in the mapping effort of the Human Genome Project (HGP). GDB's mission is to provide scientists with an encyclopedia of the human genome which is continually revised and updated to reflect the current state of scientific knowledge. Although GDB has historically focused on gene mapping, its focus will broaden as the Genome Project moves from mapping to sequence, and finally, to functional analysis.

To access the GDB, simply go to the following hyperlink: **http://www.gdb.org/**. Search "All Biological Data" by "Keyword." Type "scleroderma" (or synonyms) into the search box, and review the results. If more than one word is used in the search box, then separate each one with the word "and" or "or" (using "or" might be useful when using synonyms). This database is extremely technical as it was created for specialists. The articles are the results which are the most accessible to non-professionals and often listed under the heading "Citations." The contact names are also accessible to non-professionals.

Specialized References

The following books are specialized references written for professionals interested in scleroderma (sorted alphabetically by title, hyperlinks provide rankings, information, and reviews at Amazon.com):

- **Atlas of Clinical Dermatology** by Du Vivier; Hardcover, 3rd edition (June 3, 2002), Churchill Livingstone; ISBN: 0443072205; **http://www.amazon.com/exec/obidos/ASIN/0443072205/icongroupinterna**

- **Clinical Dermatology** by John A. Hunter, et al; Paperback, 3rd edition (June 2002), Blackwell Science Inc; ISBN: 0632059168; **http://www.amazon.com/exec/obidos/ASIN/0632059168/icongroupinterna**

- **Clinical Dermatology: A Color Guide to Diagnosis and Therapy** by Thomas P. Habif; Hardcover, 4th edition (July 15, 2002), Mosby-Year Book; ISBN: 0323013198; **http://www.amazon.com/exec/obidos/ASIN/0323013198/icongroupinterna**

- **Common Skin Diseases** by Thomas F. Poyner; Paperback - 176 pages, 1st edition (March 15, 2000), Blackwell Science Inc.; ISBN: 0632051345; **http://www.amazon.com/exec/obidos/ASIN/0071054480/icongroupinterna**

- **Dermatology (Pocket Brain)** by Kimberly N. Jones; Hardcover (March 2002); ISBN: 0967783925; **http://www.amazon.com/exec/obidos/ASIN/0967783925/icongroupinterna**

- **Dermatology for Clinicians** by Massad G. Joseph; Hardcover - 320 pages (June 5, 2002), CRC Press-Parthenon Publishers; ISBN: 1842141260; http://www.amazon.com/exec/obidos/ASIN/1842141260/icongroupinterna

- **Essential Dermatopathology** by Ronald P. Rapini; Hardcover (August 2002), Mosby-Year Book; ISBN: 0323011985; http://www.amazon.com/exec/obidos/ASIN/0323011985/icongroupinterna

- **Evidence-Based Dermatology** by Maibach; Hardcover (March 2002), B C Decker; ISBN: 1550091727; http://www.amazon.com/exec/obidos/ASIN/1550091727/icongroupinterna

- **A Multi-Cultural Atlas of Skin Conditions** by Darya Samolis, Yuri N. Perjamutrov; Paperback - 120 pages (March 19, 2002); ISBN: 1873413424; http://www.amazon.com/exec/obidos/ASIN/1873413424/icongroupinterna

- **Treatment of Skin Disease** by Mark Lebwohl, et al; Hardcover - 600 pages, 1st edition (March 27, 2002), Mosby, Inc.; ISBN: 0723431981; http://www.amazon.com/exec/obidos/ASIN/0723431981/icongroupinterna

CHAPTER 10. DISSERTATIONS ON SCLERODERMA

Overview

University researchers are active in studying almost all known diseases. The result of research is often published in the form of Doctoral or Master's dissertations. You should understand, therefore, that applied diagnostic procedures and/or therapies can take many years to develop after the thesis that proposed the new technique or approach was written.

In this chapter, we will give you a bibliography on recent dissertations relating to scleroderma. You can read about these in more detail using the Internet or your local medical library. We will also provide you with information on how to use the Internet to stay current on dissertations.

Dissertations on Scleroderma

ProQuest Digital Dissertations is the largest archive of academic dissertations available. From this archive, we have compiled the following list covering dissertations devoted to scleroderma. You will see that the information provided includes the dissertation's title, its author, and the author's institution. To read more about the following, simply use the Internet address indicated. The following covers recent dissertations dealing with scleroderma:

- **Symptom Reporting and Acid Sensitivity in Barrett's Oesophagus and Scleroderma** by Gibbons, Michael Joseph; Md from Queen's University of Belfast (northern Ireland), 2001, 240 pages
  http://wwwlib.umi.com/dissertations/fullcit/f499089

Keeping Current

As previously mentioned, an effective way to stay current on dissertations dedicated to scleroderma is to use the database called *ProQuest Digital Dissertations* via the Internet, located at the following Web address: **http://wwwlib.umi.com/dissertations.** The site allows you to freely access the last two years of citations and abstracts. Ask your medical librarian if the library has full and unlimited access to this database. From the library, you should be able to do more complete searches than with the limited 2-year access available to the general public.

PART III. APPENDICES

ABOUT PART III

Part III is a collection of appendices on general medical topics which may be of interest to patients with scleroderma and related conditions.

APPENDIX A. RESEARCHING YOUR MEDICATIONS

Overview

There are a number of sources available on new or existing medications which could be prescribed to patients with scleroderma. While a number of hard copy or CD-Rom resources are available to patients and physicians for research purposes, a more flexible method is to use Internet-based databases. In this chapter, we will begin with a general overview of medications. We will then proceed to outline official recommendations on how you should view your medications. You may also want to research medications that you are currently taking for other conditions as they may interact with medications for scleroderma. Research can give you information on the side effects, interactions, and limitations of prescription drugs used in the treatment of scleroderma. Broadly speaking, there are two sources of information on approved medications: public sources and private sources. We will emphasize free-to-use public sources.

Your Medications: The Basics[42]

The Agency for Health Care Research and Quality has published extremely useful guidelines on how you can best participate in the medication aspects of scleroderma. Taking medicines is not always as simple as swallowing a pill. It can involve many steps and decisions each day. The AHCRQ recommends that patients with scleroderma take part in treatment decisions. Do not be afraid to ask questions and talk about your concerns. By taking a moment to ask questions early, you may avoid problems later. Here are some points to cover each time a new medicine is prescribed:

- Ask about all parts of your treatment, including diet changes, exercise, and medicines.

- Ask about the risks and benefits of each medicine or other treatment you might receive.

- Ask how often you or your doctor will check for side effects from a given medication.

Do not hesitate to ask what is important to you about your medicines. You may want a medicine with the fewest side effects, or the fewest doses to take each day. You may care most about cost, or how the medicine might affect how you live or work. Or, you may want the medicine your doctor believes will work the best. Telling your doctor will help him or her select the best treatment for you.

Do not be afraid to "bother" your doctor with your concerns and questions about medications for scleroderma. You can also talk to a nurse or a pharmacist. They can help you better understand your treatment plan. Feel free to bring a friend or family member with you when you visit your doctor. Talking over your options with someone you trust can help you make better choices, especially if you are not feeling well. Specifically, ask your doctor the following:

- The name of the medicine and what it is supposed to do.

- How and when to take the medicine, how much to take, and for how long.

- What food, drinks, other medicines, or activities you should avoid while taking the medicine.

- What side effects the medicine may have, and what to do if they occur.

- If you can get a refill, and how often.

---

[42] This section is adapted from AHCRQ: **http://www.ahcpr.gov/consumer/ncpiebro.htm**.

- About any terms or directions you do not understand.

- What to do if you miss a dose.

- If there is written information you can take home (most pharmacies have information sheets on your prescription medicines; some even offer large-print or Spanish versions).

Do not forget to tell your doctor about all the medicines you are currently taking (not just those for scleroderma). This includes prescription medicines and the medicines that you buy over the counter. Then your doctor can avoid giving you a new medicine that may not work well with the medications you take now. When talking to your doctor, you may wish to prepare a list of medicines you currently take, the reason you take them, and how you take them. Be sure to include the following information for each:

- Name of medicine

- Reason taken

- Dosage

- Time(s) of day

Also include any over-the-counter medicines, such as:

- Laxatives

- Diet pills

- Vitamins

- Cold medicine

- Aspirin or other pain, headache, or fever medicine

- Cough medicine

- Allergy relief medicine

- Antacids

- Sleeping pills

- Others (include names)

Learning More about Your Medications

Because of historical investments by various organizations and the emergence of the Internet, it has become rather simple to learn about the medications your doctor has recommended for scleroderma. One such source is the United States Pharmacopeia. In 1820, eleven physicians met in Washington, D.C. to establish the first compendium of standard drugs for the United States. They called this compendium the "U.S. Pharmacopeia (USP)." Today, the USP is a non-profit organization consisting of 800 volunteer scientists, eleven elected officials, and 400 representatives of state associations and colleges of medicine and pharmacy. The USP is located in Rockville, Maryland, and its home page is located at **www.usp.org**. The USP currently provides standards for over 3,700 medications. The resulting USP DI® Advice for the Patient® can be accessed through the National Library of Medicine of the National Institutes of Health. The database is partially derived from lists of federally approved medications in the Food and Drug Administration's (FDA) Drug Approvals database.[43]

While the FDA database is rather large and difficult to navigate, the Phamacopeia is both user-friendly and free to use. It covers more than 9,000 prescription and over-the-counter medications. To access this database, simply type the following hyperlink into your Web browser: **http://www.nlm.nih.gov/medlineplus/druginformation.html**. To view examples of a given medication (brand names, category, description, preparation, proper use, precautions, side effects, etc.), simply follow the hyperlinks indicated within the United States Pharmacopoeia (USP). It is important to read the disclaimer by the USP (**http://www.nlm.nih.gov/medlineplus/drugdisclaimer.html**) before using the information provided.

Of course, we as editors cannot be certain as to what medications you are taking. Therefore, we have compiled a list of medications associated with the treatment of scleroderma. Once again, due to space limitations, we only list a sample of medications and provide hyperlinks to ample documentation (e.g. typical dosage, side effects, drug-interaction risks, etc.). The following drugs have been mentioned in the Pharmacopeia and other sources as being potentially applicable to scleroderma:

Aminobenzoate Potassium
- **Systemic - U.S. Brands:** Potaba
  http://www.nlm.nih.gov/medlineplus/druginfo/aminobenzoate
  potassiumsystemic202025.html

---

[43] Though cumbersome, the FDA database can be freely browsed at the following site: **www.fda.gov/cder/da/da.htm**.

Angiotensin-Converting Enzyme (Ace) Inhibitors
- **Systemic - U.S. Brands:** Accupril; Aceon; Altace; Capoten; Lotensin; Mavik; Monopril; Prinivil; Univasc; Vasotec 4; Zestril
http://www.nlm.nih.gov/medlineplus/druginfo/angiotensinconvertingenzymeace202044.html

Bleomycin
- **Systemic - U.S. Brands:** Blenoxane
http://www.nlm.nih.gov/medlineplus/druginfo/bleomycinsystemic202093.html

Clindamycin
- **Systemic - U.S. Brands:** Cleocin
http://www.nlm.nih.gov/medlineplus/druginfo/clindamycinsystemic202145.html
- **Topical - U.S. Brands:** Clinda-Derm
http://www.nlm.nih.gov/medlineplus/druginfo/clindamycintopical202146.html
- **Vaginal - U.S. Brands:** Cleocin
http://www.nlm.nih.gov/medlineplus/druginfo/clindamycinvaginal202700.html

Dimethyl Sulfoxide
- **Mucosal - U.S. Brands:** Rimso-50
http://www.nlm.nih.gov/medlineplus/druginfo/dimethylsulfoxidemucosal202196.html

Epoprostenol
- **Systemic - U.S. Brands:** Flolan
http://www.nlm.nih.gov/medlineplus/druginfo/epoprostenolsystemic203429.html

Erythromycin
- **Ophthalmic - U.S. Brands:** Ilotycin
http://www.nlm.nih.gov/medlineplus/druginfo/erythromycinophthalmic202220.html

Silver Sulfadiazine
- **Topical - U.S. Brands:** Silvadene; SSD; Thermazene
http://www.nlm.nih.gov/medlineplus/druginfo/silversulfadiazinetopical202521.html

Commercial Databases

In addition to the medications listed in the USP above, a number of commercial sites are available by subscription to physicians and their institutions. You may be able to access these sources from your local medical library or your doctor's office.

Reuters Health Drug Database

The Reuters Health Drug Database can be searched by keyword at the hyperlink: **http://www.reutershealth.com/frame2/drug.html**. The following medications are listed in the Reuters' database as associated with scleroderma (including those with contraindications):[44]

- **Captopril**
  http://www.reutershealth.com/atoz/html/Captopril.htm

- **Chloroquine**
  http://www.reutershealth.com/atoz/html/Chloroquine.htm

- **Colchicine**
  http://www.reutershealth.com/atoz/html/Colchicine.htm

- **Corticotropin**
  http://www.reutershealth.com/atoz/html/Corticotropin.htm

- **Corticotropin (Adrenocorticotropic hormone; ACTH)**
  http://www.reutershealth.com/atoz/html/Corticotropin_(Adrenocorticotropic_hormone;_ACTH).htm

- **Enalapril Maleate**
  http://www.reutershealth.com/atoz/html/Enalapril_Maleate.htm

Mosby's GenRx

Mosby's GenRx database (also available on CD-Rom and book format) covers 45,000 drug products including generics and international brands. It provides prescribing information, drug interactions, and patient information. Information can be obtained at the following hyperlink: **http://www.genrx.com/Mosby/PhyGenRx/group.html**.

---

[44] Adapted from *A to Z Drug Facts* by Facts and Comparisons.

Physicians Desk Reference

The Physicians Desk Reference database (also available in CD-Rom and book format) is a full-text drug database. The database is searchable by brand name, generic name or by indication. It features multiple drug interactions reports. Information can be obtained at the following hyperlink: **http://physician.pdr.net/physician/templates/en/acl/psuser_t.htm**.

Other Web Sites

A number of additional Web sites discuss drug information. As an example, you may like to look at **www.drugs.com** which reproduces the information in the Pharmacopeia as well as commercial information. You may also want to consider the Web site of the Medical Letter, Inc. which allows users to download articles on various drugs and therapeutics for a nominal fee: **http://www.medletter.com/**.

Contraindications and Interactions (Hidden Dangers)

Some of the medications mentioned in the previous discussions can be problematic for patients with scleroderma--not because they are used in the treatment process, but because of contraindications, or side effects. Medications with contraindications are those that could react with drugs used to treat scleroderma or potentially create deleterious side effects in patients with scleroderma. You should ask your physician about any contraindications, especially as these might apply to other medications that you may be taking for common ailments.

Drug-drug interactions occur when two or more drugs react with each other. This drug-drug interaction may cause you to experience an unexpected side effect. Drug interactions may make your medications less effective, cause unexpected side effects, or increase the action of a particular drug. Some drug interactions can even be harmful to you.

Be sure to read the label every time you use a nonprescription or prescription drug, and take the time to learn about drug interactions. These precautions may be critical to your health. You can reduce the risk of potentially harmful drug interactions and side effects with a little bit of knowledge and common sense.

Drug labels contain important information about ingredients, uses, warnings, and directions which you should take the time to read and understand. Labels also include warnings about possible drug interactions. Further, drug labels may change as new information becomes available. This is why it's especially important to read the label every time you use a medication. When your doctor prescribes a new drug, discuss all over-the-counter and prescription medications, dietary supplements, vitamins, botanicals, minerals and herbals you take as well as the foods you eat. Ask your pharmacist for the package insert for each prescription drug you take. The package insert provides more information about potential drug interactions.

A Final Warning

At some point, you may hear of alternative medications from friends, relatives, or in the news media. Advertisements may suggest that certain alternative drugs can produce positive results for patients with scleroderma. Exercise caution--some of these drugs may have fraudulent claims, and others may actually hurt you. The Food and Drug Administration (FDA) is the official U.S. agency charged with discovering which medications are likely to improve the health of patients with scleroderma. The FDA warns patients to watch out for[45]:

- Secret formulas (real scientists share what they know)

- Amazing breakthroughs or miracle cures (real breakthroughs don't happen very often; when they do, real scientists do not call them amazing or miracles)

- Quick, painless, or guaranteed cures

- If it sounds too good to be true, it probably isn't true.

If you have any questions about any kind of medical treatment, the FDA may have an office near you. Look for their number in the blue pages of the phone book. You can also contact the FDA through its toll-free number, 1-888-INFO-FDA (1-888-463-6332), or on the World Wide Web at **www.fda.gov**.

The following is a specific Web list relating to scleroderma; please note that any particular subject below may indicate either a therapeutic use, or a

---

[45] This section has been adapted from http://www.fda.gov/opacom/lowlit/medfraud.html.

contraindication (potential danger), and does not reflect an official recommendation:

- **General Overview**

  Dupuytren's Contracture
  Source: Healthnotes, Inc.; www.healthnotes.com
  Hyperlink:
  http://www.thedacare.org/healthnotes/Concern/Dupuytrens_Contracture.htm

  Raynaud's Phenomenon
  Source: Integrative Medicine Communications;
  www.onemedicine.com
  Hyperlink:
  http://www.drkoop.com/interactivemedicine/ConsConditions/RaynaudsPhenomenoncc.html

  Scleroderma
  Source: Integrative Medicine Communications;
  www.onemedicine.com
  Hyperlink:
  http://www.drkoop.com/InteractiveMedicine/ConsLookups/Uses/scleroderma.html

  Scleroderma
  Source: Integrative Medicine Communications;
  www.onemedicine.com
  Hyperlink:
  http://www.drkoop.com/interactivemedicine/ConsConditions/Sclerodermacc.html

  Vitiligo
  Source: Healthnotes, Inc.; www.healthnotes.com
  Hyperlink:
  http://www.thedacare.org/healthnotes/Concern/Vitiligo.htm

- **Herbs and Supplements**

   ### 5-HTP
   Alternative names: 5-Hydroxytryptophan (5-HTP)
   Source: Integrative Medicine Communications;
   www.onemedicine.com
   Hyperlink:
   http://www.drkoop.com/InteractiveMedicine/ConsSupplements/In
   teractions/5Hydroxytryptophan5HTPcs.html

   ### 5-HTP
   Source: Integrative Medicine Communications;
   www.onemedicine.com
   Hyperlink:
   http://www.drkoop.com/interactivemedicine/ConsSupplements/5
   Hydroxytryptophan5HTPcs.html

   ### 5-HTP (5-Hydroxytryptophan)
   Source: Prima Communications, Inc.
   Hyperlink: http://www.personalhealthzone.com/pg000158.html
   ### 5-Hydroxytryptophan
   Source: Healthnotes, Inc.; www.healthnotes.com
   Hyperlink: http://www.thedacare.org/healthnotes/Supp/5-
   HTP.htm

   ### 5-Hydroxytryptophan (5-HTP)
   Alternative names: 5-HTP
   Source: Integrative Medicine Communications;
   www.onemedicine.com
   Hyperlink:
   http://www.drkoop.com/InteractiveMedicine/ConsSupplements/In
   teractions/5Hydroxytryptophan5HTPcs.html

   ### 5-Hydroxytryptophan (5-HTP)
   Source: Integrative Medicine Communications;
   www.onemedicine.com
   Hyperlink:
   http://www.drkoop.com/interactivemedicine/ConsSupplements/5
   Hydroxytryptophan5HTPcs.html

Ananas comosus
Source: Integrative Medicine Communications;
www.onemedicine.com
Hyperlink:
http://www.drkoop.com/interactivemedicine/ConsSupplements/Br
omelaincs.html

B-carotene
Source: Integrative Medicine Communications;
www.onemedicine.com
Hyperlink:
http://www.drkoop.com/interactivemedicine/ConsSupplements/Be
taCarotenecs.html

Beta-Carotene
Alternative names: b-carotene, Trans-beta Carotene; Provitamin A,
Betacarotenum
Source: Integrative Medicine Communications;
www.onemedicine.com
Hyperlink:
http://www.drkoop.com/interactivemedicine/ConsSupplements/Be
taCarotenecs.html

Betacarotenum
Source: Integrative Medicine Communications;
www.onemedicine.com
Hyperlink:
http://www.drkoop.com/interactivemedicine/ConsSupplements/Be
taCarotenecs.html

Brahmi
Alternative names: Centella asiatica , Centella, March Pennywort,
Indian Pennywort, Hydrocotyle, Brahmi (Sanskrit), Luei Gong Gen
(Chinese)(Note: Gotu kola should not be confused with kola nut.)
Source: Integrative Medicine Communications;
www.onemedicine.com
Hyperlink:
http://www.drkoop.com/interactivemedicine/ConsHerbs/GotuKol
ach.html

Bromelain
Alternative names: Ananas comosus, Bromelainum
Source: Integrative Medicine Communications;
www.onemedicine.com
Hyperlink:
http://www.drkoop.com/interactivemedicine/ConsSupplements/Br
omelaincs.html

Bromelainum
Source: Integrative Medicine Communications;
www.onemedicine.com
Hyperlink:
http://www.drkoop.com/interactivemedicine/ConsSupplements/Br
omelaincs.html

Carbidopa
Source: Healthnotes, Inc.; www.healthnotes.com
Hyperlink:
http://www.thedacare.org/healthnotes/Drug/Carbidopa.htm

Carbidopa/Levodopa
Source: Healthnotes, Inc.; www.healthnotes.com
Hyperlink:
http://www.thedacare.org/healthnotes/Drug/Carbidopa_Levodopa
.htm

Centella
Alternative names: Gotu Kola; Centella asiatica (Linn.)
Source: Alternative Medicine Foundation, Inc.;
www.amfoundation.org
Hyperlink: http://www.herbmed.org/

Centella
Source: Integrative Medicine Communications;
www.onemedicine.com
Hyperlink:
http://www.drkoop.com/interactivemedicine/ConsHerbs/GotuKol
ach.html

Centella asiatica

Alternative names: Centella asiatica , Centella, March Pennywort, Indian Pennywort, Hydrocotyle, Brahmi (Sanskrit), Luei Gong Gen (Chinese)(Note: Gotu kola should not be confused with kola nut.)
Source: Integrative Medicine Communications;
www.onemedicine.com
Hyperlink:
http://www.drkoop.com/interactivemedicine/ConsHerbs/GotuKolach.html

DMSO

Source: Healthnotes, Inc.; www.healthnotes.com
Hyperlink:
http://www.thedacare.org/healthnotes/Supp/DMSO.htm

Fiber

Source: Healthnotes, Inc.; www.healthnotes.com
Hyperlink: http://www.thedacare.org/healthnotes/Supp/Fiber.htm

Gotu Kola

Alternative names: Centella asiatica
Source: Healthnotes, Inc.; www.healthnotes.com
Hyperlink:
http://www.thedacare.org/healthnotes/Herb/Gotu_Kola.htm

Gotu Kola

Alternative names: Centella asiatica , Centella, March Pennywort, Indian Pennywort, Hydrocotyle, Brahmi (Sanskrit), Luei Gong Gen (Chinese)(Note: Gotu kola should not be confused with kola nut.)
Source: Integrative Medicine Communications;
www.onemedicine.com
Hyperlink:
http://www.drkoop.com/interactivemedicine/ConsHerbs/GotuKolach.html

Gotu Kola

Source: Prima Communications, Inc.
Hyperlink: http://www.personalhealthzone.com/pg000172.html

Gotu kola
Source: WholeHealthMD.com, LLC.; www.wholehealthmd.com
Hyperlink:
http://www.wholehealthmd.com/refshelf/substances_view/0,1525,
10031,00.html

Hydrocotyle
Source: Integrative Medicine Communications;
www.onemedicine.com
Hyperlink:
http://www.drkoop.com/interactivemedicine/ConsHerbs/GotuKol
ach.html

Indian Pennywort
Source: Integrative Medicine Communications;
www.onemedicine.com
Hyperlink:
http://www.drkoop.com/interactivemedicine/ConsHerbs/GotuKol
ach.html

Levodopa/Carbidopa
Alternative names: Sinemet
Source: Prima Communications, Inc.
Hyperlink: http://www.personalhealthzone.com/pg000351.html

Marsh Pennywort
Alternative names: Centella asiatica , Centella, March Pennywort,
Indian Pennywort, Hydrocotyle, Brahmi (Sanskrit), Luei Gong Gen
(Chinese)(Note: Gotu kola should not be confused with kola nut.)
Source: Integrative Medicine Communications;
www.onemedicine.com
Hyperlink:
http://www.drkoop.com/interactivemedicine/ConsHerbs/GotuKol
ach.html

PABA
Source: Healthnotes, Inc.; www.healthnotes.com
Hyperlink:
http://www.thedacare.org/healthnotes/Supp/PABA.htm

PABA
Source: WholeHealthMD.com, LLC.; www.wholehealthmd.com
Hyperlink:
http://www.wholehealthmd.com/refshelf/substances_view/0,1525,
10049,00.html

PABA (Para-Aminobenzoic Acid)
Source: Prima Communications, Inc.
Hyperlink: http://www.personalhealthzone.com/pg000217.html
Pregnenolone
Source: Healthnotes, Inc.; www.healthnotes.com
Hyperlink:
http://www.thedacare.org/healthnotes/Supp/Pregnenolone.htm

Trans-Beta-Carotene
Source: Integrative Medicine Communications;
www.onemedicine.com
Hyperlink:
http://www.drkoop.com/interactivemedicine/ConsSupplements/Be
taCarotenecs.html

General References

In addition to the resources provided earlier in this chapter, the following general references describe medications (sorted alphabetically by title; hyperlinks provide rankings, information and reviews at Amazon.com):

- **Comprehensive Dermatologic Drug Therapy** by Stephen E. Wolverton (Editor); Paperback - 656 pages (March 15, 2001), W B Saunders Co; ISBN: 0721677282;
  http://www.amazon.com/exec/obidos/ASIN/0721677282/icongroupinterna

- **Drug Eruption Reference Manual 2000, Millennium Edition** by Jerome Z. Litt, M.D. (Editor); Paperback - 662 pages (April 15, 2000), Parthenon Pub Group; ISBN: 185070788X;
  http://www.amazon.com/exec/obidos/ASIN/185070788X/icongroupinterna

- **Pocket Guide to Medications Used in Dermatology** by Andrew J. Scheman, David L. Severson; Paperback - 230 pages, 6th edition (June 15, 1999), Lippincott Williams & Wilkins Publishers; ISBN: 0781721008;
  http://www.amazon.com/exec/obidos/ASIN/0781721008/icongroupinterna

- **Complete Guide to Prescription and Nonprescription Drugs 2001 (Complete Guide to Prescription and Nonprescription Drugs, 2001)** by H. Winter Griffith, Paperback 16th edition (2001), Medical Surveillance; ISBN: 0942447417;
  http://www.amazon.com/exec/obidos/ASIN/039952634X/icongroupinterna

- **The Essential Guide to Prescription Drugs, 2001** by James J. Rybacki, James W. Long; Paperback - 1274 pages (2001), Harper Resource; ISBN: 0060958162;
  http://www.amazon.com/exec/obidos/ASIN/0060958162/icongroupinterna

- **Handbook of Commonly Prescribed Drugs** by G. John Digregorio, Edward J. Barbieri; Paperback 16th edition (2001), Medical Surveillance; ISBN: 0942447417;
  http://www.amazon.com/exec/obidos/ASIN/0942447417/icongroupinterna

- **Johns Hopkins Complete Home Encyclopedia of Drugs 2nd ed.** by Simeon Margolis (Ed.), Johns Hopkins; Hardcover - 835 pages (2000), Rebus; ISBN: 0929661583;
  http://www.amazon.com/exec/obidos/ASIN/0929661583/icongroupinterna

- **Medical Pocket Reference: Drugs 2002** by Springhouse Paperback 1st edition (2001), Lippincott Williams & Wilkins Publishers; ISBN: 1582550964;
  http://www.amazon.com/exec/obidos/ASIN/1582550964/icongroupinterna

- **PDR** by Medical Economics Staff, Medical Economics Staff Hardcover - 3506 pages 55th edition (2000), Medical Economics Company; ISBN: 1563633752;
  http://www.amazon.com/exec/obidos/ASIN/1563633752/icongroupinterna

- **Pharmacy Simplified: A Glossary of Terms** by James Grogan; Paperback - 432 pages, 1st edition (2001), Delmar Publishers; ISBN: 0766828581;
  http://www.amazon.com/exec/obidos/ASIN/0766828581/icongroupinterna

- **Physician Federal Desk Reference** by Christine B. Fraizer; Paperback 2nd edition (2001), Medicode Inc; ISBN: 1563373971;
  http://www.amazon.com/exec/obidos/ASIN/1563373971/icongroupinterna

- **Physician's Desk Reference Supplements** Paperback - 300 pages, 53 edition (1999), ISBN: 1563632950;
  http://www.amazon.com/exec/obidos/ASIN/1563632950/icongroupinterna

Vocabulary Builder

The following vocabulary builder gives definitions of words used in this chapter that have not been defined in previous chapters:

Carbidopa: A peripheral inhibitor of dopa decarboxylase. It is given in parkinsonism along with levodopa to inhibit the conversion of levodopa to dopamine in the periphery, thereby reducing the peripheral adverse effects, increasing the amount of levodopa that reaches the central nervous system, and reducing the dose needed. It has no antiparkinson actions when given alone. [NIH]

Carotene: The general name for a group of pigments found in green, yellow, and leafy vegetables, and yellow fruits. The pigments are fat-soluble, unsaturated aliphatic hydrocarbons functioning as provitamins and are converted to vitamin A through enzymatic processes in the intestinal wall. [NIH]

Chloroquine: The prototypical antimalarial agent with a mechanism that is not well understood. It has also been used to treat rheumatoid arthritis, systemic lupus erythematosus, and in the systemic therapy of amebic liver abscesses. [NIH]

Clindamycin: An antibacterial agent that is a semisynthetic analog of lincomycin. [NIH]

Dimethyl Sulfoxide: A highly polar organic liquid, that is used widely as a chemical solvent. Because of its ability to penetrate biological membranes, it is used as a vehicle for topical application of pharmaceuticals. It is also used to protect tissue during cryopreservation. Dimethyl sulfoxide shows a range of pharmacological activity including analgesia and anti-inflammation. [NIH]

Epoprostenol: A prostaglandin that is biosynthesized enzymatically from prostaglandin endoperoxides in human vascular tissue. It is a potent inhibitor of platelet aggregation. The sodium salt has been also used to treat primary pulmonary hypertension. [NIH]

Erythromycin: A bacteriostatic antibiotic substance produced by Streptomyces erythreus. Erythromycin A is considered its major active component. In sensitive organisms, it inhibits protein synthesis by binding to 50S ribosomal subunits. This binding process inhibits peptidyl transferase activity and interferes with translocation of amino acids during translation and assembly of proteins. [NIH]

Levodopa: The naturally occurring form of dopa and the immediate precursor of dopamine. Unlike dopamine itself, it can be taken orally and crosses the blood-brain barrier. It is rapidly taken up by dopaminergic neurons and converted to dopamine. It is used for the treatment of parkinsonism and is usually given with agents that inhibit its conversion to dopamine outside of the central nervous system. [NIH]

APPENDIX B. RESEARCHING ALTERNATIVE MEDICINE

Overview

Complementary and alternative medicine (CAM) is one of the most contentious aspects of modern medical practice. You may have heard of these treatments on the radio or on television. Maybe you have seen articles written about these treatments in magazines, newspapers, or books. Perhaps your friends or doctor have mentioned alternatives.

In this chapter, we will begin by giving you a broad perspective on complementary and alternative therapies. Next, we will introduce you to official information sources on CAM relating to scleroderma. Finally, at the conclusion of this chapter, we will provide a list of readings on scleroderma from various authors. We will begin, however, with the National Center for Complementary and Alternative Medicine's (NCCAM) overview of complementary and alternative medicine.

What Is CAM?[46]

Complementary and alternative medicine (CAM) covers a broad range of healing philosophies, approaches, and therapies. Generally, it is defined as those treatments and healthcare practices which are not taught in medical schools, used in hospitals, or reimbursed by medical insurance companies. Many CAM therapies are termed "holistic," which generally means that the healthcare practitioner considers the whole person, including physical, mental, emotional, and spiritual health. Some of these therapies are also known as "preventive," which means that the practitioner educates and

---

[46] Adapted from the NCCAM: **http://nccam.nih.gov/nccam/fcp/faq/index.html#what-is**.

treats the person to prevent health problems from arising, rather than treating symptoms after problems have occurred.

People use CAM treatments and therapies in a variety of ways. Therapies are used alone (often referred to as alternative), in combination with other alternative therapies, or in addition to conventional treatment (sometimes referred to as complementary). Complementary and alternative medicine, or "integrative medicine," includes a broad range of healing philosophies, approaches, and therapies. Some approaches are consistent with physiological principles of Western medicine, while others constitute healing systems with non-Western origins. While some therapies are far outside the realm of accepted Western medical theory and practice, others are becoming established in mainstream medicine.

Complementary and alternative therapies are used in an effort to prevent illness, reduce stress, prevent or reduce side effects and symptoms, or control or cure disease. Some commonly used methods of complementary or alternative therapy include mind/body control interventions such as visualization and relaxation, manual healing including acupressure and massage, homeopathy, vitamins or herbal products, and acupuncture.

What Are the Domains of Alternative Medicine?[47]

The list of CAM practices changes continually. The reason being is that these new practices and therapies are often proved to be safe and effective, and therefore become generally accepted as "mainstream" healthcare practices. Today, CAM practices may be grouped within five major domains: (1) alternative medical systems, (2) mind-body interventions, (3) biologically-based treatments, (4) manipulative and body-based methods, and (5) energy therapies. The individual systems and treatments comprising these categories are too numerous to list in this sourcebook. Thus, only limited examples are provided within each.

Alternative Medical Systems

Alternative medical systems involve complete systems of theory and practice that have evolved independent of, and often prior to, conventional biomedical approaches. Many are traditional systems of medicine that are

---

[47] Adapted from the NCCAM: http://nccam.nih.gov/nccam/fcp/classify/index.html.

practiced by individual cultures throughout the world, including a number of venerable Asian approaches.

Traditional oriental medicine emphasizes the balance or disturbances of qi (pronounced chi) or vital energy in health and disease, respectively. Traditional oriental medicine consists of a group of techniques and methods including acupuncture, herbal medicine, oriental massage, and qi gong (a form of energy therapy). Acupuncture involves stimulating specific anatomic points in the body for therapeutic purposes, usually by puncturing the skin with a thin needle.

Ayurveda is India's traditional system of medicine. Ayurvedic medicine (meaning "science of life") is a comprehensive system of medicine that places equal emphasis on body, mind, and spirit. Ayurveda strives to restore the innate harmony of the individual. Some of the primary Ayurvedic treatments include diet, exercise, meditation, herbs, massage, exposure to sunlight, and controlled breathing.

Other traditional healing systems have been developed by the world's indigenous populations. These populations include Native American, Aboriginal, African, Middle Eastern, Tibetan, and Central and South American cultures. Homeopathy and naturopathy are also examples of complete alternative medicine systems.

Homeopathic medicine is an unconventional Western system that is based on the principle that "like cures like," i.e., that the same substance that in large doses produces the symptoms of an illness, in very minute doses cures it. Homeopathic health practitioners believe that the more dilute the remedy, the greater its potency. Therefore, they use small doses of specially prepared plant extracts and minerals to stimulate the body's defense mechanisms and healing processes in order to treat illness.

Naturopathic medicine is based on the theory that disease is a manifestation of alterations in the processes by which the body naturally heals itself and emphasizes health restoration rather than disease treatment. Naturopathic physicians employ an array of healing practices, including the following: diet and clinical nutrition, homeopathy, acupuncture, herbal medicine, hydrotherapy (the use of water in a range of temperatures and methods of applications), spinal and soft-tissue manipulation, physical therapies (such as those involving electrical currents, ultrasound, and light), therapeutic counseling, and pharmacology.

Mind-Body Interventions

Mind-body interventions employ a variety of techniques designed to facilitate the mind's capacity to affect bodily function and symptoms. Only a select group of mind-body interventions having well-documented theoretical foundations are considered CAM. For example, patient education and cognitive-behavioral approaches are now considered "mainstream." On the other hand, complementary and alternative medicine includes meditation, certain uses of hypnosis, dance, music, and art therapy, as well as prayer and mental healing.

Biological-Based Therapies

This category of CAM includes natural and biological-based practices, interventions, and products, many of which overlap with conventional medicine's use of dietary supplements. This category includes herbal, special dietary, orthomolecular, and individual biological therapies.

Herbal therapy employs an individual herb or a mixture of herbs for healing purposes. An herb is a plant or plant part that produces and contains chemical substances that act upon the body. Special diet therapies, such as those proposed by Drs. Atkins, Ornish, Pritikin, and Weil, are believed to prevent and/or control illness as well as promote health. Orthomolecular therapies aim to treat disease with varying concentrations of chemicals such as magnesium, melatonin, and mega-doses of vitamins. Biological therapies include, for example, the use of laetrile and shark cartilage to treat cancer and the use of bee pollen to treat autoimmune and inflammatory diseases.

Manipulative and Body-Based Methods

This category includes methods that are based on manipulation and/or movement of the body. For example, chiropractors focus on the relationship between structure and function, primarily pertaining to the spine, and how that relationship affects the preservation and restoration of health. Chiropractors use manipulative therapy as an integral treatment tool.

In contrast, osteopaths place particular emphasis on the musculoskeletal system and practice osteopathic manipulation. Osteopaths believe that all of the body's systems work together and that disturbances in one system may have an impact upon function elsewhere in the body. Massage therapists manipulate the soft tissues of the body to normalize those tissues.

Energy Therapies

Energy therapies focus on energy fields originating within the body (biofields) or those from other sources (electromagnetic fields). Biofield therapies are intended to affect energy fields (the existence of which is not yet experimentally proven) that surround and penetrate the human body. Some forms of energy therapy manipulate biofields by applying pressure and/or manipulating the body by placing the hands in or through these fields. Examples include Qi gong, Reiki and Therapeutic Touch.

Qi gong is a component of traditional oriental medicine that combines movement, meditation, and regulation of breathing to enhance the flow of vital energy (qi) in the body, improve blood circulation, and enhance immune function. Reiki, the Japanese word representing Universal Life Energy, is based on the belief that, by channeling spiritual energy through the practitioner, the spirit is healed and, in turn, heals the physical body. Therapeutic Touch is derived from the ancient technique of "laying-on of hands." It is based on the premises that the therapist's healing force affects the patient's recovery and that healing is promoted when the body's energies are in balance. By passing their hands over the patient, these healers identify energy imbalances.

Bioelectromagnetic-based therapies involve the unconventional use of electromagnetic fields to treat illnesses or manage pain. These therapies are often used to treat asthma, cancer, and migraine headaches. Types of electromagnetic fields which are manipulated in these therapies include pulsed fields, magnetic fields, and alternating current or direct current fields.

Can Alternatives Affect My Treatment?

A critical issue in pursuing complementary alternatives mentioned thus far is the risk that these might have undesirable interactions with your medical treatment. It becomes all the more important to speak with your doctor who can offer advice on the use of alternatives. Official sources confirm this view. Though written for women, we find that the National Women's Health Information Center's advice on pursuing alternative medicine is appropriate for patients of both genders and all ages.[48]

---

[48] Adapted from **http://www.4woman.gov/faq/alternative.htm** .

Is It Okay to Want Both Traditional and Alternative Medicine?

Should you wish to explore non-traditional types of treatment, be sure to discuss all issues concerning treatments and therapies with your healthcare provider, whether a physician or practitioner of complementary and alternative medicine. Competent healthcare management requires knowledge of both conventional and alternative therapies you are taking for the practitioner to have a complete picture of your treatment plan.

The decision to use complementary and alternative treatments is an important one. Consider before selecting an alternative therapy, the safety and effectiveness of the therapy or treatment, the expertise and qualifications of the healthcare practitioner, and the quality of delivery. These topics should be considered when selecting any practitioner or therapy.

Finding CAM References on Scleroderma

Having read the previous discussion, you may be wondering which complementary or alternative treatments might be appropriate for scleroderma. For the remainder of this chapter, we will direct you to a number of official sources which can assist you in researching studies and publications. Some of these articles are rather technical, so some patience may be required.

National Center for Complementary and Alternative Medicine

The National Center for Complementary and Alternative Medicine (NCCAM) of the National Institutes of Health (http://nccam.nih.gov) has created a link to the National Library of Medicine's databases to allow patients to search for articles that specifically relate to scleroderma and complementary medicine. To search the database, go to the following Web site: **www.nlm.nih.gov/nccam/camonpubmed.html**. Select "CAM on PubMed." Enter "scleroderma" (or synonyms) into the search box. Click "Go." The following references provide information on particular aspects of complementary and alternative medicine (CAM) that are related to scleroderma:

- **A trial of acupuncture for progressive systemic sclerosis.**
  Author(s): Maeda M, Ichiki Y, Sumi A, Mori S.

Source: J Dermatol. 1988 April; 15(2): 133-40. No Abstract Available.
http://www.ncbi.nlm.nih.gov:80/entrez/query.fcgi?cmd=Retrieve&db=
PubMed&list_uids=3049730&dopt=Abstract

- **An objective evaluation of the treatment of systemic scleroderma with disodium EDTA, pyridoxine and reserpine.**
  Author(s): Fuleihan FJ, Kurban AK, Abboud RT, Beidas-Jubran N, Farah FS.
  Source: The British Journal of Dermatology. 1968 March; 80(3): 184-9. No Abstract Available.
  http://www.ncbi.nlm.nih.gov:80/entrez/query.fcgi?cmd=Retrieve&db=
  PubMed&list_uids=4967134&dopt=Abstract

- **Behavioral treatment of Raynaud's phenomenon in scleroderma.**
  Author(s): Freedman RR, Ianni P, Wenig P.
  Source: Journal of Behavioral Medicine. 1984 December; 7(4): 343-53.
  http://www.ncbi.nlm.nih.gov:80/entrez/query.fcgi?cmd=Retrieve&db=
  PubMed&list_uids=6520866&dopt=Abstract

- **Disseminated scleroderma of a Japanese patient successfully treated with bath PUVA photochemotherapy.**
  Author(s): Aragane Y, Kawada A, Maeda A, Isogai R, Isogai N, Tezuka T.
  Source: Journal of Cutaneous Medicine and Surgery. 2001 March-April; 5(2): 135-9.
  http://www.ncbi.nlm.nih.gov:80/entrez/query.fcgi?cmd=Retrieve&db=
  PubMed&list_uids=11443486&dopt=Abstract

- **Docetaxel (Taxotere) associated scleroderma-like changes of the lower extremities. A report of three cases.**
  Author(s): Battafarano DF, Zimmerman GC, Older SA, Keeling JH, Burris HA.
  Source: Cancer. 1995 July 1; 76(1): 110-5.
  http://www.ncbi.nlm.nih.gov:80/entrez/query.fcgi?cmd=Retrieve&db=
  PubMed&list_uids=8630861&dopt=Abstract

- **Effect of ethylenediaminetetraacetic acid (EDTA) and tetrahydroxyquinone on sclerodermatous skin. Histologic and chemical studies.**
  Author(s): Keech MK, McCann DS, Boyle AJ, Pinkus H.

Source: The Journal of Investigative Dermatology. 1966 September; 47(3): 235-46. No Abstract Available.
http://www.ncbi.nlm.nih.gov:80/entrez/query.fcgi?cmd=Retrieve&db=PubMed&list_uids=4958819&dopt=Abstract

- **Effect of transcutaneous nerve stimulation on esophageal motility in patients with achalasia and scleroderma.**
  Author(s): Mearin F, Zacchi P, Armengol JR, Vilardell M, Malagelada JR.
  Source: Scandinavian Journal of Gastroenterology. 1990 October; 25(10): 1018-23.
  http://www.ncbi.nlm.nih.gov:80/entrez/query.fcgi?cmd=Retrieve&db=PubMed&list_uids=2263874&dopt=Abstract

- **Efficacy of physiatric management of linear scleroderma.**
  Author(s): Rudolph RI, Leyden JJ, Berger BJ.
  Source: Archives of Physical Medicine and Rehabilitation. 1974 September; 55(9): 428-31. No Abstract Available.
  http://www.ncbi.nlm.nih.gov:80/entrez/query.fcgi?cmd=Retrieve&db=PubMed&list_uids=4413188&dopt=Abstract

- **Inhibition of collagen production by traditional Chinese herbal medicine in scleroderma fibroblast cultures.**
  Author(s): Sheng FY, Ohta A, Yamaguchi M.
  Source: Intern Med. 1994 August; 33(8): 466-71.
  http://www.ncbi.nlm.nih.gov:80/entrez/query.fcgi?cmd=Retrieve&db=PubMed&list_uids=7803912&dopt=Abstract

- **Kinetochore structure, duplication, and distribution in mammalian cells: analysis by human autoantibodies from scleroderma patients.**
  Author(s): Brenner S, Pepper D, Berns MW, Tan E, Brinkley BR.
  Source: The Journal of Cell Biology. 1981 October; 91(1): 95-102.
  http://www.ncbi.nlm.nih.gov:80/entrez/query.fcgi?cmd=Retrieve&db=PubMed&list_uids=7298727&dopt=Abstract

- **Management of finger ulcers in scleroderma.**
  Author(s): Ward WA, Van Moore A.
  Source: The Journal of Hand Surgery. 1995 September; 20(5): 868-72.
  http://www.ncbi.nlm.nih.gov:80/entrez/query.fcgi?cmd=Retrieve&db=PubMed&list_uids=8522759&dopt=Abstract

- **Marked digital skin temperature increase mediated by thermal biofeedback in advanced scleroderma.**
  Author(s): Wilson E, Belar CD, Panush RS, Ettinger MP.
  Source: J Rheumatol. 1983 February; 10(1): 167-8. No Abstract Available.
  http://www.ncbi.nlm.nih.gov:80/entrez/query.fcgi?cmd=Retrieve&db=PubMed&list_uids=6842480&dopt=Abstract

- **Of faddism, toxic oil, and scleroderma.**
  Author(s): Berry CL.
  Source: The Journal of Pathology. 1993 August; 170(4): 419-20. No Abstract Available.
  http://www.ncbi.nlm.nih.gov:80/entrez/query.fcgi?cmd=Retrieve&db=PubMed&list_uids=8410491&dopt=Abstract

- **Physiotherapeutic viewpoints in progressive scleroderma**
  Author(s): Callies R, Danz J, Lindau P.
  Source: Z Gesamte Inn Med. 1976 January 15; 31(2): 50-1.
  http://www.ncbi.nlm.nih.gov:80/entrez/query.fcgi?cmd=Retrieve&db=PubMed&list_uids=960891&dopt=Abstract

- **Raynaud's phenomenon in scleroderma treated with hyperbaric oxygen.**
  Author(s): Dowling GB, Copeman PW, Ashfield R.
  Source: Proc R Soc Med. 1967 December; 60(12): 1268-9. No Abstract Available.
  http://www.ncbi.nlm.nih.gov:80/entrez/query.fcgi?cmd=Retrieve&db=PubMed&list_uids=6066573&dopt=Abstract

- **Remission of scleroderma during chemotherapy for lymphoma.**
  Author(s): Comer M, Harvey AR.
  Source: Annals of the Rheumatic Diseases. 1992 August; 51(8): 998-1000.
  http://www.ncbi.nlm.nih.gov:80/entrez/query.fcgi?cmd=Retrieve&db=PubMed&list_uids=1417129&dopt=Abstract

- **Scleroderma in a child after chemotherapy for cancer.**
  Author(s): Emir S, Kutluk T, Topaloglu R, Bakkaloglu A, Buyukpamukcu M.
  Source: Clin Exp Rheumatol. 2001 March-April; 19(2): 221-3.
  http://www.ncbi.nlm.nih.gov:80/entrez/query.fcgi?cmd=Retrieve&db=PubMed&list_uids=11326490&dopt=Abstract

- **Scleroderma in association with the use of docetaxel (taxotere) for breast cancer.**
  Author(s): Hassett G, Harnett P, Manolios N.
  Source: Clin Exp Rheumatol. 2001 March-April; 19(2): 197-200.
  http://www.ncbi.nlm.nih.gov:80/entrez/query.fcgi?cmd=Retrieve&db=PubMed&list_uids=11326485&dopt=Abstract

- **Scleroderma overlap syndromes.**
  Author(s): Jablonska S, Blaszczyk M.
  Source: Advances in Experimental Medicine and Biology. 1999; 455: 85-92.
  http://www.ncbi.nlm.nih.gov:80/entrez/query.fcgi?cmd=Retrieve&db=PubMed&list_uids=10599327&dopt=Abstract

- **Scleroderma. 1. Clinical features, course of illness and response to treatment in 61 cases.**
  Author(s): Barnett AJ, Coventry DA.
  Source: The Medical Journal of Australia. 1969 May 10; 1(19): 992-1001.
  No Abstract Available.
  http://www.ncbi.nlm.nih.gov:80/entrez/query.fcgi?cmd=Retrieve&db=PubMed&list_uids=4978080&dopt=Abstract

- **Scleroderma: the more you know, the more you can help.**
  Author(s): Zalac CJ.
  Source: J Pract Nurs. 1979 August; 29(8): 23-5. No Abstract Available.
  http://www.ncbi.nlm.nih.gov:80/entrez/query.fcgi?cmd=Retrieve&db=PubMed&list_uids=257011&dopt=Abstract

- **Stimulating circulation to end stasis in scleroderma.**
  Author(s): Yuan X, Li JD, Chen WJ, Li ZS, Zhu HT, Liu JW, Zhu MJ.
  Source: Chin Med J (Engl). 1981 February; 94(2): 85-93. No Abstract Available.
  http://www.ncbi.nlm.nih.gov:80/entrez/query.fcgi?cmd=Retrieve&db=PubMed&list_uids=6786844&dopt=Abstract

- **Transcutaneous electrical nerve stimulation and extensor splint in linear scleroderma knee contracture.**
  Author(s): Rizk TE, Park SJ.

Source: Archives of Physical Medicine and Rehabilitation. 1981 February; 62(2): 86-8.

http://www.ncbi.nlm.nih.gov:80/entrez/query.fcgi?cmd=Retrieve&db= PubMed&list_uids=6972203&dopt=Abstract

- **Treatment of generalized scleroderma with combined traditional Chinese and western medicine: report of 30 cases.**
  Author(s): Dexin W.
  Source: Chin Med J (Engl). 1979 June; 92(6): 427-30. No Abstract Available.
  http://www.ncbi.nlm.nih.gov:80/entrez/query.fcgi?cmd=Retrieve&db= PubMed&list_uids=110556&dopt=Abstract

- **Treatment of localised scleroderma with PUVA bath photochemotherapy.**
  Author(s): Kerscher M, Volkenandt M, Meurer M, Lehmann P, Plewig G, Rocken M.
  Source: Lancet. 1994 May 14; 343(8907): 1233. No Abstract Available.
  http://www.ncbi.nlm.nih.gov:80/entrez/query.fcgi?cmd=Retrieve&db= PubMed&list_uids=7909904&dopt=Abstract

- **Tryptophan metabolism in man (with special reference to rheumatoid arthritis and scleroderma).**
  Author(s): Houpt JB, Ogryzlo MA, Hunt M.
  Source: Seminars in Arthritis and Rheumatism. 1973; 2(4): 333-53. No Abstract Available.
  http://www.ncbi.nlm.nih.gov:80/entrez/query.fcgi?cmd=Retrieve&db= PubMed&list_uids=4267284&dopt=Abstract

- **Understanding the special needs of the patient with scleroderma.**
  Author(s): Rossiter RC.
  Source: Australian Nursing Journal (July 1993). 2000 September; 8(3): Suppl 1-4. Review. No Abstract Available.
  http://www.ncbi.nlm.nih.gov:80/entrez/query.fcgi?cmd=Retrieve&db= PubMed&list_uids=11894369&dopt=Abstract

Additional Web Resources

A number of additional Web sites offer encyclopedic information covering CAM and related topics. The following is a representative sample:

- Alternative Medicine Foundation, Inc.: **http://www.herbmed.org/**

- AOL: **http://search.aol.com/cat.adp?id=169&layer=&from=subcats**

- Chinese Medicine: **http://www.newcenturynutrition.com/**

- drkoop.com®: **http://www.drkoop.com/InteractiveMedicine/IndexC.html**

- Family Village: **http://www.familyvillage.wisc.edu/med_altn.htm**

- Google: **http://directory.google.com/Top/Health/Alternative/**

- Healthnotes: **http://www.thedacare.org/healthnotes/**

- Open Directory Project: **http://dmoz.org/Health/Alternative/**

- TPN.com: **http://www.tnp.com/**

- Yahoo.com: **http://dir.yahoo.com/Health/Alternative_Medicine/**

- WebMD®Health: **http://my.webmd.com/drugs_and_herbs**

- WellNet: **http://www.wellnet.ca/herbsa-c.htm**

- WholeHealthMD.com: **http://www.wholehealthmd.com/reflib/0,1529,,00.html**

General References

A good place to find general background information on CAM is the National Library of Medicine. It has prepared within the MEDLINEplus system an information topic page dedicated to complementary and alternative medicine. To access this page, go to the MEDLINEplus site at: **www.nlm.nih.gov/medlineplus/alternativemedicine.html.** This Web site provides a general overview of various topics and can lead to a number of general sources. The following additional references describe, in broad terms, alternative and complementary medicine (sorted alphabetically by title; hyperlinks provide rankings, information, and reviews at Amazon.com):

- **The Skin Cancer Answer** by I. William Lane, et al; Paperback - 160 pages (February 1999), Avery Penguin Putnam; ISBN: 0895298651; **http://www.amazon.com/exec/obidos/ASIN/0895298651/icongroupinterna**

- **Smart Medicine for Your Skin: A Comprehensive Guide to Understanding Conventional and Alternative Therapies to Heal Common Skin Problems** by Jeanette Jacknin, M.D.; Paperback - 414 pages (August 6, 2001), Avery Penguin Putnam; ISBN: 1583330984; http://www.amazon.com/exec/obidos/ASIN/1583330984/icongroupinterna

- **Alternative Medicine for Dummies** by James Dillard (Author); Audio Cassette, Abridged edition (1998), Harper Audio; ISBN: 0694520659; http://www.amazon.com/exec/obidos/ASIN/0694520659/icongroupinterna

- **Complementary and Alternative Medicine Secrets** by W. Kohatsu (Editor); Hardcover (2001), Hanley & Belfus; ISBN: 1560534400; http://www.amazon.com/exec/obidos/ASIN/1560534400/icongroupinterna

- **Dictionary of Alternative Medicine** by J. C. Segen; Paperback-2nd edition (2001), Appleton & Lange; ISBN: 0838516211; http://www.amazon.com/exec/obidos/ASIN/0838516211/icongroupinterna

- **Eat, Drink, and Be Healthy: The Harvard Medical School Guide to Healthy Eating** by Walter C. Willett, MD, et al; Hardcover - 352 pages (2001), Simon & Schuster; ISBN: 0684863375; http://www.amazon.com/exec/obidos/ASIN/0684863375/icongroupinterna

- **Encyclopedia of Natural Medicine, Revised 2nd Edition** by Michael T. Murray, Joseph E. Pizzorno; Paperback - 960 pages, 2nd Rev edition (1997), Prima Publishing; ISBN: 0761511571; http://www.amazon.com/exec/obidos/ASIN/0761511571/icongroupinterna

- **Integrative Medicine: An Introduction to the Art & Science of Healing** by Andrew Weil (Author); Audio Cassette, Unabridged edition (2001), Sounds True; ISBN: 1564558541; http://www.amazon.com/exec/obidos/ASIN/1564558541/icongroupinterna

- **New Encyclopedia of Herbs & Their Uses** by Deni Bown; Hardcover - 448 pages, Revised edition (2001), DK Publishing; ISBN: 078948031X; http://www.amazon.com/exec/obidos/ASIN/078948031X/icongroupinterna

- **Textbook of Complementary and Alternative Medicine** by Wayne B. Jonas; Hardcover (2003), Lippincott, Williams & Wilkins; ISBN: 0683044370; http://www.amazon.com/exec/obidos/ASIN/0683044370/icongroupinterna

For additional information on complementary and alternative medicine, ask your doctor or write to:

National Institutes of Health
National Center for Complementary and Alternative Medicine Clearinghouse
P. O. Box 8218
Silver Spring, MD 20907-8218

The following is a specific Web list relating to scleroderma; please note that any particular subject below may indicate either a therapeutic use, or a contraindication (potential danger), and does not reflect an official recommendation:

- **Vitamins**

  Provitamin A
  Source: Integrative Medicine Communications;
  www.onemedicine.com
  Hyperlink:
  http://www.drkoop.com/interactivemedicine/ConsSupplements/BetaCarotenecs.html

  Vitamin E
  Alternative names: Alpha-Tocopherol, Beta-Tocopherol, D-Alpha-Tocopherol, Delta-Tocopherol, Gamma-Tocopherol
  Source: Integrative Medicine Communications;
  www.onemedicine.com
  Hyperlink:
  http://www.drkoop.com/interactivemedicine/ConsSupplements/VitaminEcs.html

- **Minerals**

  Alpha-Tocopherol
  Source: Integrative Medicine Communications;
  www.onemedicine.com
  Hyperlink:
  http://www.drkoop.com/interactivemedicine/ConsSupplements/VitaminEcs.html

Beta-Tocopherol

Source: Integrative Medicine Communications;
www.onemedicine.com
Hyperlink:
http://www.drkoop.com/interactivemedicine/ConsSupplements/Vi
taminEcs.html

D-Alpha-Tocopherol

Source: Integrative Medicine Communications;
www.onemedicine.com
Hyperlink:
http://www.drkoop.com/interactivemedicine/ConsSupplements/Vi
taminEcs.html

Delta-Tocopherol

Source: Integrative Medicine Communications;
www.onemedicine.com
Hyperlink:
http://www.drkoop.com/interactivemedicine/ConsSupplements/Vi
taminEcs.html

Gamma-Tocopherol

Source: Integrative Medicine Communications;
www.onemedicine.com
Hyperlink:
http://www.drkoop.com/interactivemedicine/ConsSupplements/Vi
taminEcs.html

APPENDIX C. RESEARCHING NUTRITION

Overview

Since the time of Hippocrates, doctors have understood the importance of diet and nutrition to patients' health and well-being. Since then, they have accumulated an impressive archive of studies and knowledge dedicated to this subject. Based on their experience, doctors and healthcare providers may recommend particular dietary supplements to patients with scleroderma. Any dietary recommendation is based on a patient's age, body mass, gender, lifestyle, eating habits, food preferences, and health condition. It is therefore likely that different patients with scleroderma may be given different recommendations. Some recommendations may be directly related to scleroderma, while others may be more related to the patient's general health. These recommendations, themselves, may differ from what official sources recommend for the average person.

In this chapter we will begin by briefly reviewing the essentials of diet and nutrition that will broadly frame more detailed discussions of scleroderma. We will then show you how to find studies dedicated specifically to nutrition and scleroderma.

Food and Nutrition: General Principles

What Are Essential Foods?

Food is generally viewed by official sources as consisting of six basic elements: (1) fluids, (2) carbohydrates, (3) protein, (4) fats, (5) vitamins, and (6) minerals. Consuming a combination of these elements is considered to be a healthy diet:

- **Fluids** are essential to human life as 80-percent of the body is composed of water. Water is lost via urination, sweating, diarrhea, vomiting, diuretics (drugs that increase urination), caffeine, and physical exertion.

- **Carbohydrates** are the main source for human energy (thermoregulation) and the bulk of typical diets. They are mostly classified as being either simple or complex. Simple carbohydrates include sugars which are often consumed in the form of cookies, candies, or cakes. Complex carbohydrates consist of starches and dietary fibers. Starches are consumed in the form of pastas, breads, potatoes, rice, and other foods. Soluble fibers can be eaten in the form of certain vegetables, fruits, oats, and legumes. Insoluble fibers include brown rice, whole grains, certain fruits, wheat bran and legumes.

- **Proteins** are eaten to build and repair human tissues. Some foods that are high in protein are also high in fat and calories. Food sources for protein include nuts, meat, fish, cheese, and other dairy products.

- **Fats** are consumed for both energy and the absorption of certain vitamins. There are many types of fats, with many general publications recommending the intake of unsaturated fats or those low in cholesterol.

Vitamins and minerals are fundamental to human health, growth, and, in some cases, disease prevention. Most are consumed in your diet (exceptions being vitamins K and D which are produced by intestinal bacteria and sunlight on the skin, respectively). Each vitamin and mineral plays a different role in health. The following outlines essential vitamins:

- **Vitamin A** is important to the health of your eyes, hair, bones, and skin; sources of vitamin A include foods such as eggs, carrots, and cantaloupe.

- **Vitamin B^1**, also known as thiamine, is important for your nervous system and energy production; food sources for thiamine include meat, peas, fortified cereals, bread, and whole grains.

- **Vitamin B^2**, also known as riboflavin, is important for your nervous system and muscles, but is also involved in the release of proteins from nutrients; food sources for riboflavin include dairy products, leafy vegetables, meat, and eggs.

- **Vitamin B^3**, also known as niacin, is important for healthy skin and helps the body use energy; food sources for niacin include peas, peanuts, fish, and whole grains

- **Vitamin B^6**, also known as pyridoxine, is important for the regulation of cells in the nervous system and is vital for blood formation; food sources for pyridoxine include bananas, whole grains, meat, and fish.

- **Vitamin B^{12}** is vital for a healthy nervous system and for the growth of red blood cells in bone marrow; food sources for vitamin B^{12} include yeast, milk, fish, eggs, and meat.

- **Vitamin C** allows the body's immune system to fight various diseases, strengthens body tissue, and improves the body's use of iron; food sources for vitamin C include a wide variety of fruits and vegetables.

- **Vitamin D** helps the body absorb calcium which strengthens bones and teeth; food sources for vitamin D include oily fish and dairy products.

- **Vitamin E** can help protect certain organs and tissues from various degenerative diseases; food sources for vitamin E include margarine, vegetables, eggs, and fish.

- **Vitamin K** is essential for bone formation and blood clotting; common food sources for vitamin K include leafy green vegetables.

- **Folic Acid** maintains healthy cells and blood and, when taken by a pregnant woman, can prevent her fetus from developing neural tube defects; food sources for folic acid include nuts, fortified breads, leafy green vegetables, and whole grains.

It should be noted that one can overdose on certain vitamins which become toxic if consumed in excess (e.g. vitamin A, D, E and K).

Like vitamins, minerals are chemicals that are required by the body to remain in good health. Because the human body does not manufacture these chemicals internally, we obtain them from food and other dietary sources. The more important minerals include:

- **Calcium** is needed for healthy bones, teeth, and muscles, but also helps the nervous system function; food sources for calcium include dry beans, peas, eggs, and dairy products.

- **Chromium** is helpful in regulating sugar levels in blood; food sources for chromium include egg yolks, raw sugar, cheese, nuts, beets, whole grains, and meat.

- **Fluoride** is used by the body to help prevent tooth decay and to reinforce bone strength; sources of fluoride include drinking water and certain brands of toothpaste.

- **Iodine** helps regulate the body's use of energy by synthesizing into the hormone thyroxine; food sources include leafy green vegetables, nuts, egg yolks, and red meat.

- **Iron** helps maintain muscles and the formation of red blood cells and certain proteins; food sources for iron include meat, dairy products, eggs, and leafy green vegetables.

- **Magnesium** is important for the production of DNA, as well as for healthy teeth, bones, muscles, and nerves; food sources for magnesium include dried fruit, dark green vegetables, nuts, and seafood.

- **Phosphorous** is used by the body to work with calcium to form bones and teeth; food sources for phosphorous include eggs, meat, cereals, and dairy products.

- **Selenium** primarily helps maintain normal heart and liver functions; food sources for selenium include wholegrain cereals, fish, meat, and dairy products.

- **Zinc** helps wounds heal, the formation of sperm, and encourage rapid growth and energy; food sources include dried beans, shellfish, eggs, and nuts.

The United States government periodically publishes recommended diets and consumption levels of the various elements of food. Again, your doctor may encourage deviations from the average official recommendation based on your specific condition. To learn more about basic dietary guidelines, visit the Web site: **http://www.health.gov/dietaryguidelines/**. Based on these guidelines, many foods are required to list the nutrition levels on the food's packaging. Labeling Requirements are listed at the following site maintained by the Food and Drug Administration: **http://www.cfsan.fda.gov/~dms/lab-cons.html**. When interpreting these requirements, the government recommends that consumers become familiar with the following abbreviations before reading FDA literature:[49]

- **DVs (Daily Values):** A new dietary reference term that will appear on the food label. It is made up of two sets of references, DRVs and RDIs.

- **DRVs (Daily Reference Values):** A set of dietary references that applies to fat, saturated fat, cholesterol, carbohydrate, protein, fiber, sodium, and potassium.

---

[49] Adapted from the FDA: **http://www.fda.gov/fdac/special/foodlabel/dvs.html**.

- **RDIs (Reference Daily Intakes):** A set of dietary references based on the Recommended Dietary Allowances for essential vitamins and minerals and, in selected groups, protein. The name "RDI" replaces the term "U.S. RDA."

- **RDAs (Recommended Dietary Allowances):** A set of estimated nutrient allowances established by the National Academy of Sciences. It is updated periodically to reflect current scientific knowledge.

What Are Dietary Supplements?[50]

Dietary supplements are widely available through many commercial sources, including health food stores, grocery stores, pharmacies, and by mail. Dietary supplements are provided in many forms including tablets, capsules, powders, gel-tabs, extracts, and liquids. Historically in the United States, the most prevalent type of dietary supplement was a multivitamin/mineral tablet or capsule that was available in pharmacies, either by prescription or "over the counter." Supplements containing strictly herbal preparations were less widely available. Currently in the United States, a wide array of supplement products are available, including vitamin, mineral, other nutrients, and botanical supplements as well as ingredients and extracts of animal and plant origin.

The Office of Dietary Supplements (ODS) of the National Institutes of Health is the official agency of the United States which has the expressed goal of acquiring "new knowledge to help prevent, detect, diagnose, and treat disease and disability, from the rarest genetic disorder to the common cold."[51] According to the ODS, dietary supplements can have an important impact on the prevention and management of disease and on the maintenance of health.[52] The ODS notes that considerable research on the effects of dietary supplements has been conducted in Asia and Europe where

---

[50] This discussion has been adapted from the NIH:
http://ods.od.nih.gov/whatare/whatare.html.

[51] Contact: The Office of Dietary Supplements, National Institutes of Health, Building 31, Room 1B29, 31 Center Drive, MSC 2086, Bethesda, Maryland 20892-2086, Tel: (301) 435-2920, Fax: (301) 480-1845, E-mail: **ods@nih.gov.**

[52] Adapted from **http://ods.od.nih.gov/about/about.html.** The Dietary Supplement Health and Education Act defines dietary supplements as "a product (other than tobacco) intended to supplement the diet that bears or contains one or more of the following dietary ingredients: a vitamin, mineral, amino acid, herb or other botanical; or a dietary substance for use to supplement the diet by increasing the total dietary intake; or a concentrate, metabolite, constituent, extract, or combination of any ingredient described above; and intended for ingestion in the form of a capsule, powder, softgel, or gelcap, and not represented as a conventional food or as a sole item of a meal or the diet."

the use of plant products, in particular, has a long tradition. However, the overwhelming majority of supplements have not been studied scientifically. To explore the role of dietary supplements in the improvement of health care, the ODS plans, organizes, and supports conferences, workshops, and symposia on scientific topics related to dietary supplements. The ODS often works in conjunction with other NIH Institutes and Centers, other government agencies, professional organizations, and public advocacy groups.

To learn more about official information on dietary supplements, visit the ODS site at **http://ods.od.nih.gov/whatare/whatare.html**. Or contact:

> The Office of Dietary Supplements
> National Institutes of Health
> Building 31, Room 1B29
> 31 Center Drive, MSC 2086
> Bethesda, Maryland 20892-2086
> Tel: (301) 435-2920
> Fax: (301) 480-1845
> E-mail: ods@nih.gov

Finding Studies on Scleroderma

The NIH maintains an office dedicated to patient nutrition and diet. The National Institutes of Health's Office of Dietary Supplements (ODS) offers a searchable bibliographic database called the IBIDS (International Bibliographic Information on Dietary Supplements). The IBIDS contains over 460,000 scientific citations and summaries about dietary supplements and nutrition as well as references to published international, scientific literature on dietary supplements such as vitamins, minerals, and botanicals.[53] IBIDS is available to the public free of charge through the ODS Internet page: **http://ods.od.nih.gov/databases/ibids.html**.

After entering the search area, you have three choices: (1) IBIDS Consumer Database, (2) Full IBIDS Database, or (3) Peer Reviewed Citations Only. We recommend that you start with the Consumer Database. While you may not find references for the topics that are of most interest to you, check back

---

[53] Adapted from http://ods.od.nih.gov. IBIDS is produced by the Office of Dietary Supplements (ODS) at the National Institutes of Health to assist the public, healthcare providers, educators, and researchers in locating credible, scientific information on dietary supplements. IBIDS was developed and will be maintained through an interagency partnership with the Food and Nutrition Information Center of the National Agricultural Library, U.S. Department of Agriculture.

periodically as this database is frequently updated. More studies can be found by searching the Full IBIDS Database. Healthcare professionals and researchers generally use the third option, which lists peer-reviewed citations. In all cases, we suggest that you take advantage of the "Advanced Search" option that allows you to retrieve up to 100 fully explained references in a comprehensive format. Type "scleroderma" (or synonyms) into the search box. To narrow the search, you can also select the "Title" field.

The following information is typical of that found when using the "Full IBIDS Database" when searching using "scleroderma" (or a synonym):

- **A 15-year prospective study of treatment of rapidly progressive systemic sclerosis with D-penicillamine [see comment]**
  Author(s): Department of Medicine, Jefferson Medical College, Thomas Jefferson University, Philadelphia, PA 19107.
  Source: Jimenez, S A Sigal, S H J-Rheumatol. 1991 October; 18(10): 1496-503 0315-162X

- **A double-blind placebo-controlled trial of antioxidant therapy in limited cutaneous systemic sclerosis.**
  Author(s): University of Manchester Rheumatic Diseases Centre, Hope Hospital, Salford, UK. aherrick@fs1.ho.man.ac.uk
  Source: Herrick, A L Hollis, S Schofield, D Rieley, F Blann, A Griffin, K Moore, T Braganza, J M Jayson, M I Clin-Exp-Rheumatol. 2000 May-June; 18(3): 349-56 0392-856X

- **A randomised, double-blind study of cicaprost, an oral prostacyclin analogue, in the treatment of Raynaud's phenomenon secondary to systemic sclerosis.**
  Author(s): University Department of Medicine, Ninewells Hospital and Medical School, Dundee, Scotland.
  Source: Lau, C S Belch, J J Madhok, R Cappell, H Herrick, A Jayson, M Thompson, J M Clin-Exp-Rheumatol. 1993 Jan-February; 11(1): 35-40 0392-856X

- **Abnormal lymphocyte function in scleroderma: a study on identical twins.**
  Source: Dustoor, M M McInerney, M M Mazanec, D J Cathcart, M K Clin-Immunol-Immunopathol. 1987 July; 44(1): 20-30 0090-1229

- **Acute effects of nebulised epoprostenol in pulmonary hypertension due to systemic sclerosis.**
  Author(s): Department of Respiratory Medicine, Royal Sunderland Hospital, U.K. parames@fhs.mcmaster.ca

Source: Parameswaran, K Purcell, I Farrer, M Holland, C Taylor, I K Keaney, N P Respir-Med. 1999 February; 93(2): 75-8 0954-6111

- **Acute estrogen administration can reverse cold-induced coronary Raynaud's phenomenon in systemic sclerosis.**
Author(s): Department of Clinical Therapeutics, Alexandra University Hospital, Athens, Greece.
Source: Lekakis, J Mavrikakis, M Emmanuel, M Prassopoulos, V Papamichael, C Moulopoulou, D Ziaga, A Kostamis, P Moulopoulos, S Clin-Exp-Rheumatol. 1996 Jul-August; 14(4): 421-4 0392-856X

- **Antiphospholipid syndrome associated with progressive systemic sclerosis.**
Author(s): Department of Dermatology, Yonsei University College of Medicine, Seoul, Korea.
Source: Chun, W H Bang, D Lee, S K J-Dermatol. 1996 May; 23(5): 347-51 0385-2407

- **Benign breast disease in systemic sclerosis (SSc). A case-control study.**
Author(s): Rheumatic Diseases Unit, Ottawa General Hospital, University of Ottawa, Ontario, Canada.
Source: McKendry, R J Cyr, M Dale, P Clin-Exp-Rheumatol. 1992 May-June; 10(3): 235-9 0392-856X

- **Bioavailability of D-penicillamine in relation to gastrointestinal involvement of generalized scleroderma.**
Source: Ammitzboll, T Hendel, L Kreuzig, F Asboe Hansen, G Scand-J-Rheumatol. 1987; 16(2): 121-6 0300-9742

- **Calcium-channel blockers for Raynaud's phenomenon in systemic sclerosis.**
Author(s): University of Western Ontario, London, Canada.
Source: Thompson, A E Shea, B Welch, V Fenlon, D Pope, J E Arthritis-Rheum. 2001 August; 44(8): 1841-7 0004-3591

- **Chromosome abnormalities in peripheral lymphocytes from patients with progressive systemic sclerosis.**
Author(s): Department of Medicine and Physical Therapy, Faculty of Medicine, University of Tokyo, Japan.
Source: Takeuchi, F Nakano, K Yamada, H Kosuge, E Hirai, M Maeda, H Moroi, Y Rheumatol-Int. 1993; 12(6): 243-6 0172-8172

- **Clinical trials for the treatment of systemic sclerosis/scleroderma.**
Author(s): Department of Medicine, University of Illinois at Chicago College of Medicine, Chicago, IL, USA.
Source: Varga, J Ponor, I Curr-Rheumatol-Repage 1999 October; 1(1): 13-4 1523-3774

- **Collagen in the extracellular matrix of cultured scleroderma skin fibroblasts: changes related to ascorbic acid-treatment.**
  Author(s): Department of Medical Biochemistry, University of Turku, Finland.
  Source: Heino, J Kahari, V M Jaakkola, S Peltonen, J Matrix. 1989 January; 9(1): 34-9 0934-8832

- **Comparative assessment of the effects of vasodilators on peripheral vascular reactivity in patients with systemic scleroderma and Raynaud's phenomenon: color Doppler flow imaging study.**
  Author(s): Department of Radiology, Balcali Hospital, Cukurova University, Medical School, Adana, Turkey.
  Source: Aikimbaev, K S Oguz, M Ozbek, S Demirtas, M Birand, A Batyraliev, T Angiology. 1996 May; 47(5): 475-80 0003-3197

- **Cytokine production in scleroderma patients: effects of therapy with either iloprost or nifedipine.**
  Author(s): Institute of Internal Medicine, Infectious Diseases and Immunopathology, IRCCS Ospedale Maggiore di Milano, Italy.
  Source: Della Bella, S Molteni, M Mascagni, B Zulian, C Compasso, S Scorza, R Clin-Exp-Rheumatol. 1997 Mar-April; 15(2): 135-41 0392-856X

Federal Resources on Nutrition

In addition to the IBIDS, the United States Department of Health and Human Services (HHS) and the United States Department of Agriculture (USDA) provide many sources of information on general nutrition and health. Recommended resources include:

- healthfinder®, HHS's gateway to health information, including diet and nutrition:
  http://www.healthfinder.gov/scripts/SearchContext.asp?topic=238&page=0

- The United States Department of Agriculture's Web site dedicated to nutrition information: **www.nutrition.gov**

- The Food and Drug Administration's Web site for federal food safety information: **www.foodsafety.gov**

- The National Action Plan on Overweight and Obesity sponsored by the United States Surgeon General:
  http://www.surgeongeneral.gov/topics/obesity/

- The Center for Food Safety and Applied Nutrition has an Internet site sponsored by the Food and Drug Administration and the Department of Health and Human Services: **http://vm.cfsan.fda.gov/**

- Center for Nutrition Policy and Promotion sponsored by the United States Department of Agriculture: **http://www.usda.gov/cnpp/**

- Food and Nutrition Information Center, National Agricultural Library sponsored by the United States Department of Agriculture: **http://www.nal.usda.gov/fnic/**

- Food and Nutrition Service sponsored by the United States Department of Agriculture: **http://www.fns.usda.gov/fns/**

Additional Web Resources

A number of additional Web sites offer encyclopedic information covering food and nutrition. The following is a representative sample:

- AOL: **http://search.aol.com/cat.adp?id=174&layer=&from=subcats**

- Family Village: **http://www.familyvillage.wisc.edu/med_nutrition.html**

- Google: **http://directory.google.com/Top/Health/Nutrition/**

- Healthnotes: **http://www.thedacare.org/healthnotes/**

- Open Directory Project: **http://dmoz.org/Health/Nutrition/**

- Yahoo.com: **http://dir.yahoo.com/Health/Nutrition/**

- WebMD®Health: **http://my.webmd.com/nutrition**

- WholeHealthMD.com: **http://www.wholehealthmd.com/reflib/0,1529,,00.html**

Vocabulary Builder

The following vocabulary builder defines words used in the references in this chapter that have not been defined in previous chapters:

Acitretin: An oral retinoid effective in the treatment of psoriasis. It is the major metabolite of etretinate with the advantage of a much shorter half-life when compared with etretinate. [NIH]

Antioxidant: One of many widely used synthetic or natural substances added to a product to prevent or delay its deterioration by action of oxygen in the air. Rubber, paints, vegetable oils, and prepared foods commonly contain antioxidants. [EU]

Bioavailability: The degree to which a drug or other substance becomes available to the target tissue after administration. [EU]

Capsules: Hard or soft soluble containers used for the oral administration of medicine. [NIH]

Carbohydrate: An aldehyde or ketone derivative of a polyhydric alcohol, particularly of the pentahydric and hexahydric alcohols. They are so named because the hydrogen and oxygen are usually in the proportion to form water, $(CH2O)n$. The most important carbohydrates are the starches, sugars, celluloses, and gums. They are classified into mono-, di-, tri-, poly- and heterosaccharides. [EU]

Cholesterol: The principal sterol of all higher animals, distributed in body tissues, especially the brain and spinal cord, and in animal fats and oils. [NIH]

Coronary: Encircling in the manner of a crown; a term applied to vessels; nerves, ligaments, etc. The term usually denotes the arteries that supply the heart muscle and, by extension, a pathologic involvement of them. [EU]

Iodine: A nonmetallic element of the halogen group that is represented by the atomic symbol I, atomic number 53, and atomic weight of 126.90. It is a nutritionally essential element, especially important in thyroid hormone synthesis. In solution, it has anti-infective properties and is used topically. [NIH]

Niacin: Water-soluble vitamin of the B complex occurring in various animal and plant tissues. Required by the body for the formation of coenzymes NAD and NADP. Has pellagra-curative, vasodilating, and antilipemic properties. [NIH]

Overdose: 1. to administer an excessive dose. 2. an excessive dose. [EU]

Riboflavin: Nutritional factor found in milk, eggs, malted barley, liver, kidney, heart, and leafy vegetables. The richest natural source is yeast. It occurs in the free form only in the retina of the eye, in whey, and in urine; its principal forms in tissues and cells are as FMN and FAD. [NIH]

Selenium: An element with the atomic symbol Se, atomic number 34, and atomic weight 78.96. It is an essential micronutrient for mammals and other animals but is toxic in large amounts. Selenium protects intracellular structures against oxidative damage. It is an essential component of glutathione peroxidase. [NIH]

Thyroxine: An amino acid of the thyroid gland which exerts a stimulating effect on thyroid metabolism. [NIH]

Tomography: The recording of internal body images at a predetermined plane by means of the tomograph; called also body section roentgenography. [EU]

APPENDIX D. FINDING MEDICAL LIBRARIES

Overview

At a medical library you can find medical texts and reference books, consumer health publications, specialty newspapers and magazines, as well as medical journals. In this Appendix, we show you how to quickly find a medical library in your area.

Preparation

Before going to the library, highlight the references mentioned in this sourcebook that you find interesting. Focus on those items that are not available via the Internet, and ask the reference librarian for help with your search. He or she may know of additional resources that could be helpful to you. Most importantly, your local public library and medical libraries have Interlibrary Loan programs with the National Library of Medicine (NLM), one of the largest medical collections in the world. According to the NLM, most of the literature in the general and historical collections of the National Library of Medicine is available on interlibrary loan to any library. NLM's interlibrary loan services are only available to libraries. If you would like to access NLM medical literature, then visit a library in your area that can request the publications for you.[54]

---

[54] Adapted from the NLM: http://www.nlm.nih.gov/psd/cas/interlibrary.html.

Finding a Local Medical Library

The quickest method to locate medical libraries is to use the Internet-based directory published by the National Network of Libraries of Medicine (NN/LM). This network includes 4626 members and affiliates that provide many services to librarians, health professionals, and the public. To find a library in your area, simply visit **http://nnlm.gov/members/adv.html** or call 1-800-338-7657.

Medical Libraries Open to the Public

In addition to the NN/LM, the National Library of Medicine (NLM) lists a number of libraries that are generally open to the public and have reference facilities. The following is the NLM's list plus hyperlinks to each library Web site. These Web pages can provide information on hours of operation and other restrictions. The list below is a small sample of libraries recommended by the National Library of Medicine (sorted alphabetically by name of the U.S. state or Canadian province where the library is located):[55]

- **Alabama:** Health InfoNet of Jefferson County (Jefferson County Library Cooperative, Lister Hill Library of the Health Sciences), **http://www.uab.edu/infonet/**

- **Alabama:** Richard M. Scrushy Library (American Sports Medicine Institute), **http://www.asmi.org/LIBRARY.HTM**

- **Arizona:** Samaritan Regional Medical Center: The Learning Center (Samaritan Health System, Phoenix, Arizona), **http://www.samaritan.edu/library/bannerlibs.htm**

- **California:** Kris Kelly Health Information Center (St. Joseph Health System), **http://www.humboldt1.com/~kkhic/index.html**

- **California:** Community Health Library of Los Gatos (Community Health Library of Los Gatos), **http://www.healthlib.org/orgresources.html**

- **California:** Consumer Health Program and Services (CHIPS) (County of Los Angeles Public Library, Los Angeles County Harbor-UCLA Medical Center Library) - Carson, CA, **http://www.colapublib.org/services/chips.html**

- **California:** Gateway Health Library (Sutter Gould Medical Foundation)

- **California:** Health Library (Stanford University Medical Center), **http://www-med.stanford.edu/healthlibrary/**

---

[55] Abstracted from **http://www.nlm.nih.gov/medlineplus/libraries.html**.

- **California:** Patient Education Resource Center - Health Information and Resources (University of California, San Francisco), http://sfghdean.ucsf.edu/barnett/PERC/default.asp

- **California:** Redwood Health Library (Petaluma Health Care District), http://www.phcd.org/rdwdlib.html

- **California:** San José PlaneTree Health Library, http://planetreesanjose.org/

- **California:** Sutter Resource Library (Sutter Hospitals Foundation), http://go.sutterhealth.org/comm/resc-library/sac-resources.html

- **California:** University of California, Davis. Health Sciences Libraries

- **California:** ValleyCare Health Library & Ryan Comer Cancer Resource Center (ValleyCare Health System), http://www.valleycare.com/library.html

- **California:** Washington Community Health Resource Library (Washington Community Health Resource Library), http://www.healthlibrary.org/

- **Colorado:** William V. Gervasini Memorial Library (Exempla Healthcare), http://www.exempla.org/conslib.htm

- **Connecticut:** Hartford Hospital Health Science Libraries (Hartford Hospital), http://www.harthosp.org/library/

- **Connecticut:** Healthnet: Connecticut Consumer Health Information Center (University of Connecticut Health Center, Lyman Maynard Stowe Library), http://library.uchc.edu/departm/hnet/

- **Connecticut:** Waterbury Hospital Health Center Library (Waterbury Hospital), http://www.waterburyhospital.com/library/consumer.shtml

- **Delaware:** Consumer Health Library (Christiana Care Health System, Eugene du Pont Preventive Medicine & Rehabilitation Institute), http://www.christianacare.org/health_guide/health_guide_pmri_health _info.cfm

- **Delaware:** Lewis B. Flinn Library (Delaware Academy of Medicine), http://www.delamed.org/chls.html

- **Georgia:** Family Resource Library (Medical College of Georgia), http://cmc.mcg.edu/kids_families/fam_resources/fam_res_lib/frl.htm

- **Georgia:** Health Resource Center (Medical Center of Central Georgia), http://www.mccg.org/hrc/hrchome.asp

- **Hawaii:** Hawaii Medical Library: Consumer Health Information Service (Hawaii Medical Library), http://hml.org/CHIS/

- **Idaho:** DeArmond Consumer Health Library (Kootenai Medical Center), http://www.nicon.org/DeArmond/index.htm

- **Illinois:** Health Learning Center of Northwestern Memorial Hospital (Northwestern Memorial Hospital, Health Learning Center), http://www.nmh.org/health_info/hlc.html

- **Illinois:** Medical Library (OSF Saint Francis Medical Center), http://www.osfsaintfrancis.org/general/library/

- **Kentucky:** Medical Library - Services for Patients, Families, Students & the Public (Central Baptist Hospital), http://www.centralbap.com/education/community/library.htm

- **Kentucky:** University of Kentucky - Health Information Library (University of Kentucky, Chandler Medical Center, Health Information Library), http://www.mc.uky.edu/PatientEd/

- **Louisiana:** Alton Ochsner Medical Foundation Library (Alton Ochsner Medical Foundation), http://www.ochsner.org/library/

- **Louisiana:** Louisiana State University Health Sciences Center Medical Library-Shreveport, http://lib-sh.lsuhsc.edu/

- **Maine:** Franklin Memorial Hospital Medical Library (Franklin Memorial Hospital), http://www.fchn.org/fmh/lib.htm

- **Maine:** Gerrish-True Health Sciences Library (Central Maine Medical Center), http://www.cmmc.org/library/library.html

- **Maine:** Hadley Parrot Health Science Library (Eastern Maine Healthcare), http://www.emh.org/hll/hpl/guide.htm

- **Maine:** Maine Medical Center Library (Maine Medical Center), http://www.mmc.org/library/

- **Maine:** Parkview Hospital, http://www.parkviewhospital.org/communit.htm#Library

- **Maine:** Southern Maine Medical Center Health Sciences Library (Southern Maine Medical Center), http://www.smmc.org/services/service.php3?choice=10

- **Maine:** Stephens Memorial Hospital Health Information Library (Western Maine Health), http://www.wmhcc.com/hil_frame.html

- **Manitoba, Canada:** Consumer & Patient Health Information Service (University of Manitoba Libraries), http://www.umanitoba.ca/libraries/units/health/reference/chis.html

- **Manitoba, Canada:** J.W. Crane Memorial Library (Deer Lodge Centre), http://www.deerlodge.mb.ca/library/libraryservices.shtml

- **Maryland:** Health Information Center at the Wheaton Regional Library (Montgomery County, Md., Dept. of Public Libraries, Wheaton Regional Library), **http://www.mont.lib.md.us/healthinfo/hic.asp**

- **Massachusetts:** Baystate Medical Center Library (Baystate Health System), **http://www.baystatehealth.com/1024/**

- **Massachusetts:** Boston University Medical Center Alumni Medical Library (Boston University Medical Center), **http://med-libwww.bu.edu/library/lib.html**

- **Massachusetts:** Lowell General Hospital Health Sciences Library (Lowell General Hospital), **http://www.lowellgeneral.org/library/HomePageLinks/WWW.htm**

- **Massachusetts:** Paul E. Woodard Health Sciences Library (New England Baptist Hospital), **http://www.nebh.org/health_lib.asp**

- **Massachusetts:** St. Luke's Hospital Health Sciences Library (St. Luke's Hospital), **http://www.southcoast.org/library/**

- **Massachusetts:** Treadwell Library Consumer Health Reference Center (Massachusetts General Hospital), **http://www.mgh.harvard.edu/library/chrcindex.html**

- **Massachusetts:** UMass HealthNet (University of Massachusetts Medical School), **http://healthnet.umassmed.edu/**

- **Michigan:** Botsford General Hospital Library - Consumer Health (Botsford General Hospital, Library & Internet Services), **http://www.botsfordlibrary.org/consumer.htm**

- **Michigan:** Helen DeRoy Medical Library (Providence Hospital and Medical Centers), **http://www.providence-hospital.org/library/**

- **Michigan:** Marquette General Hospital - Consumer Health Library (Marquette General Hospital, Health Information Center), **http://www.mgh.org/center.html**

- **Michigan:** Patient Education Resouce Center - University of Michigan Cancer Center (University of Michigan Comprehensive Cancer Center), **http://www.cancer.med.umich.edu/learn/leares.htm**

- **Michigan:** Sladen Library & Center for Health Information Resources - Consumer Health Information, **http://www.sladen.hfhs.org/library/consumer/index.html**

- **Montana:** Center for Health Information (St. Patrick Hospital and Health Sciences Center), **http://www.saintpatrick.org/chi/librarydetail.php3?ID=41**

- **National:** Consumer Health Library Directory (Medical Library Association, Consumer and Patient Health Information Section), http://caphis.mlanet.org/directory/index.html

- **National:** National Network of Libraries of Medicine (National Library of Medicine) - provides library services for health professionals in the United States who do not have access to a medical library, http://nnlm.gov/

- **National:** NN/LM List of Libraries Serving the Public (National Network of Libraries of Medicine), http://nnlm.gov/members/

- **Nevada:** Health Science Library, West Charleston Library (Las Vegas Clark County Library District), http://www.lvccld.org/special_collections/medical/index.htm

- **New Hampshire:** Dartmouth Biomedical Libraries (Dartmouth College Library), http://www.dartmouth.edu/~biomed/resources.htmld/conshealth.htmld/

- **New Jersey:** Consumer Health Library (Rahway Hospital), http://www.rahwayhospital.com/library.htm

- **New Jersey:** Dr. Walter Phillips Health Sciences Library (Englewood Hospital and Medical Center), http://www.englewoodhospital.com/links/index.htm

- **New Jersey:** Meland Foundation (Englewood Hospital and Medical Center), http://www.geocities.com/ResearchTriangle/9360/

- **New York:** Choices in Health Information (New York Public Library) - NLM Consumer Pilot Project participant, http://www.nypl.org/branch/health/links.html

- **New York:** Health Information Center (Upstate Medical University, State University of New York), http://www.upstate.edu/library/hic/

- **New York:** Health Sciences Library (Long Island Jewish Medical Center), http://www.lij.edu/library/library.html

- **New York:** ViaHealth Medical Library (Rochester General Hospital), http://www.nyam.org/library/

- **Ohio:** Consumer Health Library (Akron General Medical Center, Medical & Consumer Health Library), http://www.akrongeneral.org/hwlibrary.htm

- **Oklahoma:** Saint Francis Health System Patient/Family Resource Center (Saint Francis Health System), http://www.sfh-tulsa.com/patientfamilycenter/default.asp

- **Oregon:** Planetree Health Resource Center (Mid-Columbia Medical Center), **http://www.mcmc.net/phrc/**

- **Pennsylvania:** Community Health Information Library (Milton S. Hershey Medical Center), **http://www.hmc.psu.edu/commhealth/**

- **Pennsylvania:** Community Health Resource Library (Geisinger Medical Center), **http://www.geisinger.edu/education/commlib.shtml**

- **Pennsylvania:** HealthInfo Library (Moses Taylor Hospital), **http://www.mth.org/healthwellness.html**

- **Pennsylvania:** Hopwood Library (University of Pittsburgh, Health Sciences Library System), **http://www.hsls.pitt.edu/chi/hhrcinfo.html**

- **Pennsylvania:** Koop Community Health Information Center (College of Physicians of Philadelphia), **http://www.collphyphil.org/kooppg1.shtml**

- **Pennsylvania:** Learning Resources Center - Medical Library (Susquehanna Health System), **http://www.shscares.org/services/lrc/index.asp**

- **Pennsylvania:** Medical Library (UPMC Health System), **http://www.upmc.edu/passavant/library.htm**

- **Quebec, Canada:** Medical Library (Montreal General Hospital), **http://ww2.mcgill.ca/mghlib/**

- **South Dakota:** Rapid City Regional Hospital - Health Information Center (Rapid City Regional Hospital, Health Information Center), **http://www.rcrh.org/education/LibraryResourcesConsumers.htm**

- **Texas:** Houston HealthWays (Houston Academy of Medicine-Texas Medical Center Library), **http://hhw.library.tmc.edu/**

- **Texas:** Matustik Family Resource Center (Cook Children's Health Care System), **http://www.cookchildrens.com/Matustik_Library.html**

- **Washington:** Community Health Library (Kittitas Valley Community Hospital), **http://www.kvch.com/**

- **Washington:** Southwest Washington Medical Center Library (Southwest Washington Medical Center), **http://www.swmedctr.com/Home/**

APPENDIX E. YOUR RIGHTS AND INSURANCE

Overview

Any patient with scleroderma faces a series of issues related more to the healthcare industry than to the medical condition itself. This appendix covers two important topics in this regard: your rights and responsibilities as a patient, and how to get the most out of your medical insurance plan.

Your Rights as a Patient

The President's Advisory Commission on Consumer Protection and Quality in the Healthcare Industry has created the following summary of your rights as a patient.[56]

Information Disclosure

Consumers have the right to receive accurate, easily understood information. Some consumers require assistance in making informed decisions about health plans, health professionals, and healthcare facilities. Such information includes:

- *Health plans.* Covered benefits, cost-sharing, and procedures for resolving complaints, licensure, certification, and accreditation status, comparable measures of quality and consumer satisfaction, provider network composition, the procedures that govern access to specialists and emergency services, and care management information.

---

[56]Adapted from Consumer Bill of Rights and Responsibilities: http://www.hcqualitycommission.gov/press/cbor.html#head1.

- *Health professionals.* Education, board certification, and recertification, years of practice, experience performing certain procedures, and comparable measures of quality and consumer satisfaction.

- *Healthcare facilities.* Experience in performing certain procedures and services, accreditation status, comparable measures of quality, worker, and consumer satisfaction, and procedures for resolving complaints.

- *Consumer assistance programs.* Programs must be carefully structured to promote consumer confidence and to work cooperatively with health plans, providers, payers, and regulators. Desirable characteristics of such programs are sponsorship that ensures accountability to the interests of consumers and stable, adequate funding.

Choice of Providers and Plans

Consumers have the right to a choice of healthcare providers that is sufficient to ensure access to appropriate high-quality healthcare. To ensure such choice, the Commission recommends the following:

- *Provider network adequacy.* All health plan networks should provide access to sufficient numbers and types of providers to assure that all covered services will be accessible without unreasonable delay -- including access to emergency services 24 hours a day and 7 days a week. If a health plan has an insufficient number or type of providers to provide a covered benefit with the appropriate degree of specialization, the plan should ensure that the consumer obtains the benefit outside the network at no greater cost than if the benefit were obtained from participating providers.

- *Women's health services.* Women should be able to choose a qualified provider offered by a plan -- such as gynecologists, certified nurse midwives, and other qualified healthcare providers -- for the provision of covered care necessary to provide routine and preventative women's healthcare services.

- *Access to specialists.* Consumers with complex or serious medical conditions who require frequent specialty care should have direct access to a qualified specialist of their choice within a plan's network of providers. Authorizations, when required, should be for an adequate number of direct access visits under an approved treatment plan.

- *Transitional care.* Consumers who are undergoing a course of treatment for a chronic or disabling condition (or who are in the second or third trimester of a pregnancy) at the time they involuntarily change health plans or at a time when a provider is terminated by a plan for other than cause should be able to continue seeing their current specialty providers for up to 90 days (or through completion of postpartum care) to allow for transition of care.

- *Choice of health plans.* Public and private group purchasers should, wherever feasible, offer consumers a choice of high-quality health insurance plans.

Access to Emergency Services

Consumers have the right to access emergency healthcare services when and where the need arises. Health plans should provide payment when a consumer presents to an emergency department with acute symptoms of sufficient severity--including severe pain--such that a "prudent layperson" could reasonably expect the absence of medical attention to result in placing that consumer's health in serious jeopardy, serious impairment to bodily functions, or serious dysfunction of any bodily organ or part.

Participation in Treatment Decisions

Consumers have the right and responsibility to fully participate in all decisions related to their healthcare. Consumers who are unable to fully participate in treatment decisions have the right to be represented by parents, guardians, family members, or other conservators. Physicians and other health professionals should:

- Provide patients with sufficient information and opportunity to decide among treatment options consistent with the informed consent process.

- Discuss all treatment options with a patient in a culturally competent manner, including the option of no treatment at all.

- Ensure that persons with disabilities have effective communications with members of the health system in making such decisions.

- Discuss all current treatments a consumer may be undergoing.

- Discuss all risks, benefits, and consequences to treatment or nontreatment.

- Give patients the opportunity to refuse treatment and to express preferences about future treatment decisions.

- Discuss the use of advance directives -- both living wills and durable powers of attorney for healthcare -- with patients and their designated family members.

- Abide by the decisions made by their patients and/or their designated representatives consistent with the informed consent process.

Health plans, health providers, and healthcare facilities should:

- Disclose to consumers factors -- such as methods of compensation, ownership of or interest in healthcare facilities, or matters of conscience -- that could influence advice or treatment decisions.

- Assure that provider contracts do not contain any so-called "gag clauses" or other contractual mechanisms that restrict healthcare providers' ability to communicate with and advise patients about medically necessary treatment options.

- Be prohibited from penalizing or seeking retribution against healthcare professionals or other health workers for advocating on behalf of their patients.

Respect and Nondiscrimination

Consumers have the right to considerate, respectful care from all members of the healthcare industry at all times and under all circumstances. An environment of mutual respect is essential to maintain a quality healthcare system. To assure that right, the Commission recommends the following:

- Consumers must not be discriminated against in the delivery of healthcare services consistent with the benefits covered in their policy, or as required by law, based on race, ethnicity, national origin, religion, sex, age, mental or physical disability, sexual orientation, genetic information, or source of payment.

- Consumers eligible for coverage under the terms and conditions of a health plan or program, or as required by law, must not be discriminated against in marketing and enrollment practices based on race, ethnicity, national origin, religion, sex, age, mental or physical disability, sexual orientation, genetic information, or source of payment.

Confidentiality of Health Information

Consumers have the right to communicate with healthcare providers in confidence and to have the confidentiality of their individually identifiable healthcare information protected. Consumers also have the right to review and copy their own medical records and request amendments to their records.

Complaints and Appeals

Consumers have the right to a fair and efficient process for resolving differences with their health plans, healthcare providers, and the institutions that serve them, including a rigorous system of internal review and an independent system of external review. A free copy of the Patient's Bill of Rights is available from the American Hospital Association.[57]

Patient Responsibilities

Treatment is a two-way street between you and your healthcare providers. To underscore the importance of finance in modern healthcare as well as your responsibility for the financial aspects of your care, the President's Advisory Commission on Consumer Protection and Quality in the Healthcare Industry has proposed that patients understand the following "Consumer Responsibilities."[58] In a healthcare system that protects consumers' rights, it is reasonable to expect and encourage consumers to assume certain responsibilities. Greater individual involvement by the consumer in his or her care increases the likelihood of achieving the best outcome and helps support a quality-oriented, cost-conscious environment. Such responsibilities include:

- Take responsibility for maximizing healthy habits such as exercising, not smoking, and eating a healthy diet.

- Work collaboratively with healthcare providers in developing and carrying out agreed-upon treatment plans.

- Disclose relevant information and clearly communicate wants and needs.

- Use your health insurance plan's internal complaint and appeal processes to address your concerns.

- Avoid knowingly spreading disease.

---

[57] To order your free copy of the Patient's Bill of Rights, telephone 312-422-3000 or visit the American Hospital Association's Web site: http://www.aha.org. Click on "Resource Center," go to "Search" at bottom of page, and then type in "Patient's Bill of Rights." The Patient's Bill of Rights is also available from Fax on Demand, at 312-422-2020, document number 471124.

[58] Adapted from http://www.hcqualitycommission.gov/press/cbor.html#head1.

- Recognize the reality of risks, the limits of the medical science, and the human fallibility of the healthcare professional.

- Be aware of a healthcare provider's obligation to be reasonably efficient and equitable in providing care to other patients and the community.

- Become knowledgeable about your health plan's coverage and options (when available) including all covered benefits, limitations, and exclusions, rules regarding use of network providers, coverage and referral rules, appropriate processes to secure additional information, and the process to appeal coverage decisions.

- Show respect for other patients and health workers.

- Make a good-faith effort to meet financial obligations.

- Abide by administrative and operational procedures of health plans, healthcare providers, and Government health benefit programs.

Choosing an Insurance Plan

There are a number of official government agencies that help consumers understand their healthcare insurance choices.[59] The U.S. Department of Labor, in particular, recommends ten ways to make your health benefits choices work best for you.[60]

1. Your options are important. There are many different types of health benefit plans. Find out which one your employer offers, then check out the plan, or plans, offered. Your employer's human resource office, the health plan administrator, or your union can provide information to help you match your needs and preferences with the available plans. The more information you have, the better your healthcare decisions will be.

2. Reviewing the benefits available. Do the plans offered cover preventive care, well-baby care, vision or dental care? Are there deductibles? Answers to these questions can help determine the out-of-pocket expenses you may face. Matching your needs and those of your family members will result in the best possible benefits. Cheapest may not always be best. Your goal is high quality health benefits.

---

[59] More information about quality across programs is provided at the following AHRQ Web site:
http://www.ahrq.gov/consumer/qntascii/qnthplan.htm .
[60] Adapted from the Department of Labor:
http://www.dol.gov/dol/pwba/public/pubs/health/top10-text.html.

3. Look for quality. The quality of healthcare services varies, but quality can be measured. You should consider the quality of healthcare in deciding among the healthcare plans or options available to you. Not all health plans, doctors, hospitals and other providers give the highest quality care. Fortunately, there is quality information you can use right now to help you compare your healthcare choices. Find out how you can measure quality. Consult the U.S. Department of Health and Human Services publication "Your Guide to Choosing Quality Health Care" on the Internet at **www.ahcpr.gov/consumer**.

4. Your plan's summary plan description (SPD) provides a wealth of information. Your health plan administrator can provide you with a copy of your plan's SPD. It outlines your benefits and your legal rights under the Employee Retirement Income Security Act (ERISA), the federal law that protects your health benefits. It should contain information about the coverage of dependents, what services will require a co-pay, and the circumstances under which your employer can change or terminate a health benefits plan. Save the SPD and all other health plan brochures and documents, along with memos or correspondence from your employer relating to health benefits.

5. Assess your benefit coverage as your family status changes. Marriage, divorce, childbirth or adoption, and the death of a spouse are all life events that may signal a need to change your health benefits. You, your spouse and dependent children may be eligible for a special enrollment period under provisions of the Health Insurance Portability and Accountability Act (HIPAA). Even without life-changing events, the information provided by your employer should tell you how you can change benefits or switch plans, if more than one plan is offered. If your spouse's employer also offers a health benefits package, consider coordinating both plans for maximum coverage.

6. Changing jobs and other life events can affect your health benefits. Under the Consolidated Omnibus Budget Reconciliation Act (COBRA), you, your covered spouse, and your dependent children may be eligible to purchase extended health coverage under your employer's plan if you lose your job, change employers, get divorced, or upon occurrence of certain other events. Coverage can range from 18 to 36 months depending on your situation. COBRA applies to most employers with 20 or more workers and requires your plan to notify you of your rights. Most plans require eligible individuals to make their COBRA election within 60 days of the plan's notice. Be sure to follow up with your plan sponsor if you don't receive notice, and make sure you respond within the allotted time.

7. HIPAA can also help if you are changing jobs, particularly if you have a medical condition. HIPAA generally limits pre-existing condition exclusions to a maximum of 12 months (18 months for late enrollees). HIPAA also requires this maximum period to be reduced by the length of time you had prior "creditable coverage." You should receive a certificate documenting your prior creditable coverage from your old plan when coverage ends.

8. Plan for retirement. Before you retire, find out what health benefits, if any, extend to you and your spouse during your retirement years. Consult with your employer's human resources office, your union, the plan administrator, and check your SPD. Make sure there is no conflicting information among these sources about the benefits you will receive or the circumstances under which they can change or be eliminated. With this information in hand, you can make other important choices, like finding out if you are eligible for Medicare and Medigap insurance coverage.

9. Know how to file an appeal if your health benefits claim is denied. Understand how your plan handles grievances and where to make appeals of the plan's decisions. Keep records and copies of correspondence. Check your health benefits package and your SPD to determine who is responsible for handling problems with benefit claims. Contact PWBA for customer service assistance if you are unable to obtain a response to your complaint.

10. You can take steps to improve the quality of the healthcare and the health benefits you receive. Look for and use things like Quality Reports and Accreditation Reports whenever you can. Quality reports may contain consumer ratings -- how satisfied consumers are with the doctors in their plan, for instance-- and clinical performance measures -- how well a healthcare organization prevents and treats illness. Accreditation reports provide information on how accredited organizations meet national standards, and often include clinical performance measures. Look for these quality measures whenever possible. Consult "Your Guide to Choosing Quality Health Care" on the Internet at **www.ahcpr.gov/consumer**.

Medicare and Medicaid

Illness strikes both rich and poor families. For low-income families, Medicaid is available to defer the costs of treatment. The Health Care Financing Administration (HCFA) administers Medicare, the nation's largest health insurance program, which covers 39 million Americans. In the following pages, you will learn the basics about Medicare insurance as well as useful contact information on how to find more in-depth information about Medicaid.[61]

Who is Eligible for Medicare?

Generally, you are eligible for Medicare if you or your spouse worked for at least 10 years in Medicare-covered employment and you are 65 years old and a citizen or permanent resident of the United States. You might also qualify for coverage if you are under age 65 but have a disability or End-Stage Renal disease (permanent kidney failure requiring dialysis or transplant). Here are some simple guidelines:

You can get Part A at age 65 without having to pay premiums if:

- You are already receiving retirement benefits from Social Security or the Railroad Retirement Board.

- You are eligible to receive Social Security or Railroad benefits but have not yet filed for them.

- You or your spouse had Medicare-covered government employment.

If you are under 65, you can get Part A without having to pay premiums if:

- You have received Social Security or Railroad Retirement Board disability benefit for 24 months.

- You are a kidney dialysis or kidney transplant patient.

Medicare has two parts:

- Part A (Hospital Insurance). Most people do not have to pay for Part A.

- Part B (Medical Insurance). Most people pay monthly for Part B.

Part A (Hospital Insurance)

Helps Pay For: Inpatient hospital care, care in critical access hospitals (small facilities that give limited outpatient and inpatient services to people in rural areas) and skilled nursing facilities, hospice care, and some home healthcare.

---

[61] This section has been adapted from the Official U.S. Site for Medicare Information: **http://www.medicare.gov/Basics/Overview.asp**.

Cost: Most people get Part A automatically when they turn age 65. You do not have to pay a monthly payment called a premium for Part A because you or a spouse paid Medicare taxes while you were working.

If you (or your spouse) did not pay Medicare taxes while you were working and you are age 65 or older, you still may be able to buy Part A. If you are not sure you have Part A, look on your red, white, and blue Medicare card. It will show "Hospital Part A" on the lower left corner of the card. You can also call the Social Security Administration toll free at 1-800-772-1213 or call your local Social Security office for more information about buying Part A. If you get benefits from the Railroad Retirement Board, call your local RRB office or 1-800-808-0772. For more information, call your Fiscal Intermediary about Part A bills and services. The phone number for the Fiscal Intermediary office in your area can be obtained from the following Web site: **http://www.medicare.gov/Contacts/home.asp**.

Part B (Medical Insurance)

Helps Pay For: Doctors, services, outpatient hospital care, and some other medical services that Part A does not cover, such as the services of physical and occupational therapists, and some home healthcare. Part B helps pay for covered services and supplies when they are medically necessary.

Cost: As of 2001, you pay the Medicare Part B premium of $50.00 per month. In some cases this amount may be higher if you did not choose Part B when you first became eligible at age 65. The cost of Part B may go up 10% for each 12-month period that you were eligible for Part B but declined coverage, except in special cases. You will have to pay the extra 10% cost for the rest of your life.

Enrolling in Part B is your choice. You can sign up for Part B anytime during a 7-month period that begins 3 months before you turn 65. Visit your local Social Security office, or call the Social Security Administration at 1-800-772-1213 to sign up. If you choose to enroll in Part B, the premium is usually taken out of your monthly Social Security, Railroad Retirement, or Civil Service Retirement payment. If you do not receive any of the above payments, Medicare sends you a bill for your part B premium every 3 months. You should receive your Medicare premium bill in the mail by the 10th of the month. If you do not, call the Social Security Administration at 1-800-772-1213, or your local Social Security office. If you get benefits from the Railroad Retirement Board, call your local RRB office or 1-800-808-0772. For more information, call your Medicare carrier about bills and services. The phone number for the Medicare carrier in your area can be found at the following Web site: **http://www.medicare.gov/Contacts/home.asp**. You may have choices in how you get your healthcare including the Original Medicare Plan, Medicare Managed Care Plans (like HMOs), and Medicare Private Fee-for-Service Plans.

Medicaid

Medicaid is a joint federal and state program that helps pay medical costs for some people with low incomes and limited resources. Medicaid programs vary from state to state. People on Medicaid may also get coverage for nursing home care and outpatient prescription drugs which are not covered by Medicare. You can find more information about Medicaid on the HCFA.gov Web site at **http://www.hcfa.gov/medicaid/medicaid.htm**.

States also have programs that pay some or all of Medicare's premiums and may also pay Medicare deductibles and coinsurance for certain people who have Medicare and a low income. To qualify, you must have:

- Part A (Hospital Insurance),

- Assets, such as bank accounts, stocks, and bonds that are not more than $4,000 for a single person, or $6,000 for a couple, and

- A monthly income that is below certain limits.

For more information on these programs, look at the Medicare Savings Programs brochure, **http://www.medicare.gov/Library/PDFNavigation/PDFInterim.asp?Language=English&Type=Pub&PubID=10126**. There are also Prescription Drug Assistance Programs available. Find information on these programs which offer discounts or free medications to individuals in need at **http://www.medicare.gov/Prescription/Home.asp**.

NORD's Medication Assistance Programs

Finally, the National Organization for Rare Disorders, Inc. (NORD) administers medication programs sponsored by humanitarian-minded pharmaceutical and biotechnology companies to help uninsured or under-insured individuals secure life-saving or life-sustaining drugs.[62] NORD

---

62 Adapted from NORD: **http://www.rarediseases.org/cgi-bin/nord/progserv#patient?id=rPIzL9oD&mv_pc=30**.

programs ensure that certain vital drugs are available "to those individuals whose income is too high to qualify for Medicaid but too low to pay for their prescribed medications." The program has standards for fairness, equity, and unbiased eligibility. It currently covers some 14 programs for nine pharmaceutical companies. NORD also offers early access programs for investigational new drugs (IND) under the approved "Treatment INDs" programs of the Food and Drug Administration (FDA). In these programs, a limited number of individuals can receive investigational drugs that have yet to be approved by the FDA. These programs are generally designed for rare diseases or disorders. For more information, visit **www.rarediseases.org**.

Additional Resources

In addition to the references already listed in this chapter, you may need more information on health insurance, hospitals, or the healthcare system in general. The NIH has set up an excellent guidance Web site that addresses these and other issues. Topics include:[63]

- Health Insurance:
  http://www.nlm.nih.gov/medlineplus/healthinsurance.html

- Health Statistics:
  http://www.nlm.nih.gov/medlineplus/healthstatistics.html

- HMO and Managed Care:
  http://www.nlm.nih.gov/medlineplus/managedcare.html

- Hospice Care: **http://www.nlm.nih.gov/medlineplus/hospicecare.html**

- Medicaid: **http://www.nlm.nih.gov/medlineplus/medicaid.html**

- Medicare: **http://www.nlm.nih.gov/medlineplus/medicare.html**

- Nursing Homes and Long-term Care:
  http://www.nlm.nih.gov/medlineplus/nursinghomes.html

- Patient's Rights, Confidentiality, Informed Consent, Ombudsman Programs, Privacy and Patient Issues:
  http://www.nlm.nih.gov/medlineplus/patientissues.html

- Veteran's Health, Persian Gulf War, Gulf War Syndrome, Agent Orange:
  http://www.nlm.nih.gov/medlineplus/veteranshealth.html

---

[63] You can access this information at:
http://www.nlm.nih.gov/medlineplus/healthsystem.html.

Vocabulary Builder

Cardiovascular: Pertaining to the heart and blood vessels. [EU]

Dyspnea: Difficult or labored breathing. [NIH]

Hypopigmentation: A condition caused by a deficiency in melanin formation or a loss of pre-existing melanin or melanocytes. It can be complete or partial and may result from trauma, inflammation, and certain infections. [NIH]

Pruritus: 1. itching; an unpleasant cutaneous sensation that provokes the desire to rub or scratch the skin to obtain relief. 2. any of various conditions marked by itching, the specific site or type being indicated by a modifying term. [EU]

ONLINE GLOSSARIES

The Internet provides access to a number of free-to-use medical dictionaries and glossaries. The National Library of Medicine has compiled the following list of online dictionaries:

- ADAM Medical Encyclopedia (A.D.A.M., Inc.), comprehensive medical reference: **http://www.nlm.nih.gov/medlineplus/encyclopedia.html**

- MedicineNet.com Medical Dictionary (MedicineNet, Inc.): **http://www.medterms.com/Script/Main/hp.asp**

- Merriam-Webster Medical Dictionary (Inteli-Health, Inc.): **http://www.intelihealth.com/IH/**

- Multilingual Glossary of Technical and Popular Medical Terms in Eight European Languages (European Commission) - Danish, Dutch, English, French, German, Italian, Portuguese, and Spanish: **http://allserv.rug.ac.be/~rvdstich/eugloss/welcome.html**

- On-line Medical Dictionary (CancerWEB): **http://www.graylab.ac.uk/omd/**

- Technology Glossary (National Library of Medicine) - Health Care Technology: **http://www.nlm.nih.gov/nichsr/ta101/ta10108.htm**

- Terms and Definitions (Office of Rare Diseases): **http://rarediseases.info.nih.gov/ord/glossary_a-e.html**

Beyond these, MEDLINEplus contains a very user-friendly encyclopedia covering every aspect of medicine (licensed from A.D.A.M., Inc.). The ADAM Medical Encyclopedia Web site address is **http://www.nlm.nih.gov/medlineplus/encyclopedia.html**. ADAM is also available on commercial Web sites such as Web MD (**http://my.webmd.com/adam/asset/adam_disease_articles/a_to_z/a**) and drkoop.com (**http://www.drkoop.com/**). Topics of interest can be researched by using keywords before continuing elsewhere, as these basic definitions and concepts will be useful in more advanced areas of research. You may choose to print various pages specifically relating to scleroderma and keep them on file. The NIH, in particular, suggests that patients with scleroderma visit the following Web sites in the ADAM Medical Encyclopedia:

- **Basic Guidelines for Scleroderma**

  Scleroderma - resources
  Web site:
  http://www.nlm.nih.gov/medlineplus/ency/article/002195.htm

  Systemic sclerosis (scleroderma)
  Web site:
  http://www.nlm.nih.gov/medlineplus/ency/article/000429.htm

- **Signs & Symptoms for Scleroderma**

  Blanching
  Web site:
  http://www.nlm.nih.gov/medlineplus/ency/article/003249.htm

  Bloating
  Web site:
  http://www.nlm.nih.gov/medlineplus/ency/article/003123.htm

  Constipation
  Web site:
  http://www.nlm.nih.gov/medlineplus/ency/article/003125.htm

  Diarrhea
  Web site:
  http://www.nlm.nih.gov/medlineplus/ency/article/003126.htm

  Difficulty swallowing
  Web site:
  http://www.nlm.nih.gov/medlineplus/ency/article/003115.htm

  Dysphagia
  Web site:
  http://www.nlm.nih.gov/medlineplus/ency/article/003115.htm

  Dyspnea
  Web site:
  http://www.nlm.nih.gov/medlineplus/ency/article/003075.htm

Eye burning, itching and discharge
Web site:
http://www.nlm.nih.gov/medlineplus/ency/article/003034.htm

Hair loss
Web site:
http://www.nlm.nih.gov/medlineplus/ency/article/003246.htm

Heartburn
Web site:
http://www.nlm.nih.gov/medlineplus/ency/article/003114.htm

Hypopigmentation
Web site:
http://www.nlm.nih.gov/medlineplus/ency/article/003224.htm

Joint pain
Web site:
http://www.nlm.nih.gov/medlineplus/ency/article/003261.htm

Lung disease
Web site:
http://www.nlm.nih.gov/medlineplus/ency/article/000066.htm

Muscle weakness
Web site:
http://www.nlm.nih.gov/medlineplus/ency/article/003174.htm

Nausea and vomiting
Web site:
http://www.nlm.nih.gov/medlineplus/ency/article/003117.htm

Pruritus
Web site:
http://www.nlm.nih.gov/medlineplus/ency/article/003217.htm

Shortness of breath
Web site:
http://www.nlm.nih.gov/medlineplus/ency/article/003075.htm

Skin, abnormally dark or light
Web site:
http://www.nlm.nih.gov/medlineplus/ency/article/003242.htm

Stress
Web site:
http://www.nlm.nih.gov/medlineplus/ency/article/003211.htm

Swelling
Web site:
http://www.nlm.nih.gov/medlineplus/ency/article/003103.htm

Telangiectasia
Web site:
http://www.nlm.nih.gov/medlineplus/ency/article/003284.htm

Vomiting
Web site:
http://www.nlm.nih.gov/medlineplus/ency/article/003117.htm

Weakness
Web site:
http://www.nlm.nih.gov/medlineplus/ency/article/003174.htm

Weight loss
Web site:
http://www.nlm.nih.gov/medlineplus/ency/article/003107.htm

Wheezing
Web site:
http://www.nlm.nih.gov/medlineplus/ency/article/003070.htm

Wrist pain
Web site:
http://www.nlm.nih.gov/medlineplus/ency/article/003175.htm

- **Diagnostics and Tests for Scleroderma**

  ACE levels
  Web site:
  http://www.nlm.nih.gov/medlineplus/ency/article/003567.htm

ANA
Web site:
http://www.nlm.nih.gov/medlineplus/ency/article/003535.htm

Antinuclear antibody
Web site:
http://www.nlm.nih.gov/medlineplus/ency/article/003535.htm

Biopsy
Web site:
http://www.nlm.nih.gov/medlineplus/ency/article/003416.htm

Chest X-ray
Web site:
http://www.nlm.nih.gov/medlineplus/ency/article/003804.htm

CT
Web site:
http://www.nlm.nih.gov/medlineplus/ency/article/003330.htm

Esophageal manometry
Web site:
http://www.nlm.nih.gov/medlineplus/ency/article/003884.htm

ESR
Web site:
http://www.nlm.nih.gov/medlineplus/ency/article/003638.htm

Febrile/cold agglutinins
Web site:
http://www.nlm.nih.gov/medlineplus/ency/article/003549.htm

LE cell test
Web site:
http://www.nlm.nih.gov/medlineplus/ency/article/003635.htm

Lung scan
Web site:
http://www.nlm.nih.gov/medlineplus/ency/article/003824.htm

Pulmonary function
Web site:
http://www.nlm.nih.gov/medlineplus/ency/article/003443.htm

Rheumatoid factor
Web site:
http://www.nlm.nih.gov/medlineplus/ency/article/003548.htm

Skin biopsy
Web site:
http://www.nlm.nih.gov/medlineplus/ency/article/003840.htm

Urinalysis
Web site:
http://www.nlm.nih.gov/medlineplus/ency/article/003579.htm

X-ray
Web site:
http://www.nlm.nih.gov/medlineplus/ency/article/003337.htm

- **Background Topics for Scleroderma**

Cardiovascular
Web site:
http://www.nlm.nih.gov/medlineplus/ency/article/002310.htm

Incidence
Web site:
http://www.nlm.nih.gov/medlineplus/ency/article/002387.htm

Support group
Web site:
http://www.nlm.nih.gov/medlineplus/ency/article/002150.htm

Systemic
Web site:
http://www.nlm.nih.gov/medlineplus/ency/article/002294.htm

Online Dictionary Directories

The following are additional online directories compiled by the National Library of Medicine, including a number of specialized medical dictionaries and glossaries:

- Medical Dictionaries: Medical & Biological (World Health Organization): **http://www.who.int/hlt/virtuallibrary/English/diction.htm#Medical**

- MEL-Michigan Electronic Library List of Online Health and Medical Dictionaries (Michigan Electronic Library): **http://mel.lib.mi.us/health/health-dictionaries.html**

- Patient Education: Glossaries (DMOZ Open Directory Project): **http://dmoz.org/Health/Education/Patient_Education/Glossaries/**

- Web of Online Dictionaries (Bucknell University): **http://www.yourdictionary.com/diction5.html#medicine**

SCLERODERMA GLOSSARY

The following is a complete glossary of terms used in this sourcebook. The definitions are derived from official public sources including the National Institutes of Health [NIH] and the European Union [EU]. After this glossary, we list a number of additional hardbound and electronic glossaries and dictionaries that you may wish to consult.

Aberrant: Wandering or deviating from the usual or normal course. [EU]

Acetaminophen: Analgesic antipyretic derivative of acetanilide. It has weak anti-inflammatory properties and is used as a common analgesic, but may cause liver, blood cell, and kidney damage. [NIH]

Acitretin: An oral retinoid effective in the treatment of psoriasis. It is the major metabolite of etretinate with the advantage of a much shorter half-life when compared with etretinate. [NIH]

Acrodermatitis: Inflammation involving the skin of the extremities, especially the hands and feet. Several forms are known, some idiopathic and some hereditary. The infantile form is called Gianotti-Crosti syndrome. [NIH]

Adjuvant: A substance which aids another, such as an auxiliary remedy; in immunology, nonspecific stimulator (e.g., BCG vaccine) of the immune response. [EU]

Alimentary: Pertaining to food or nutritive material, or to the organs of digestion. [EU]

Alleles: Mutually exclusive forms of the same gene, occupying the same locus on homologous chromosomes, and governing the same biochemical and developmental process. [NIH]

Anemia: A reduction in the number of circulating erythrocytes or in the quantity of hemoglobin. [NIH]

Angioedema: A vascular reaction involving the deep dermis or subcutaneous or submucal tissues, representing localized edema caused by dilatation and increased permeability of the capillaries, and characterized by development of giant wheals. [EU]

Ankle: That part of the lower limb directly above the foot. [NIH]

Anorectal: Pertaining to the anus and rectum or to the junction region between the two. [EU]

Antibiotic: A chemical substance produced by a microorganism which has the capacity, in dilute solutions, to inhibit the growth of or to kill other microorganisms. Antibiotics that are sufficiently nontoxic to the host are used as chemotherapeutic agents in the treatment of infectious diseases of man, animals and plants. [EU]

Antibody: An immunoglobulin molecule that has a specific amino acid sequence by virtue of which it interacts only with the antigen that induced its synthesis in cells of the lymphoid series (especially plasma cells), or with antigen closely related to it. Antibodies are classified according to their ode of action as agglutinins, bacteriolysins, haemolysins, opsonins, precipitins, etc. [EU]

Anticoagulants: Agents that prevent blood clotting. Naturally occurring agents in the blood are included only when they are used as drugs. [NIH]

Antidepressant: An agent that stimulates the mood of a depressed patient, including tricyclic antidepressants and monoamine oxidase inhibitors. [EU]

Antigen: Any substance which is capable, under appropriate conditions, of inducing a specific immune response and of reacting with the products of that response, that is, with specific antibody or specifically sensitized T-lymphocytes, or both. Antigens may be soluble substances, such as toxins and foreign proteins, or particulate, such as bacteria and tissue cells; however, only the portion of the protein or polysaccharide molecule known as the antigenic determinant (q.v.) combines with antibody or a specific receptor on a lymphocyte. Abbreviated Ag. [EU]

Antihistamine: A drug that counteracts the action of histamine. The antihistamines are of two types. The conventional ones, as those used in allergies, block the H1 histamine receptors, whereas the others block the H2 receptors. Called also antihistaminic. [EU]

Antimicrobial: Killing microorganisms, or suppressing their multiplication or growth. [EU]

Antioxidant: One of many widely used synthetic or natural substances added to a product to prevent or delay its deterioration by action of oxygen in the air. Rubber, paints, vegetable oils, and prepared foods commonly contain antioxidants. [EU]

Antipruritic: Relieving or preventing itching. [EU]

Anxiety: The unpleasant emotional state consisting of psychophysiological responses to anticipation of unreal or imagined danger, ostensibly resulting from unrecognized intrapsychic conflict. Physiological concomitants include increased heart rate, altered respiration rate, sweating, trembling, weakness, and fatigue; psychological concomitants include feelings of impending danger, powerlessness, apprehension, and tension. [EU]

Arginine: An essential amino acid that is physiologically active in the L-form. [NIH]

Arrhythmia: Any variation from the normal rhythm of the heart beat, including sinus arrhythmia, premature beat, heart block, atrial fibrillation, atrial flutter, pulsus alternans, and paroxysmal tachycardia. [EU]

Arteries: The vessels carrying blood away from the heart. [NIH]

Aspiration: The act of inhaling. [EU]

Assay: Determination of the amount of a particular constituent of a mixture, or of the biological or pharmacological potency of a drug. [EU]

Atrophy: A wasting away; a diminution in the size of a cell, tissue, organ, or part. [EU]

Autoantigens: Endogenous tissue constituents that have the ability to interact with autoantibodies and cause an immune response. [NIH]

Autoimmunity: Process whereby the immune system reacts against the body's own tissues. Autoimmunity may produce or be caused by autoimmune diseases. [NIH]

Bacteria: Unicellular prokaryotic microorganisms which generally possess rigid cell walls, multiply by cell division, and exhibit three principal forms: round or coccal, rodlike or bacillary, and spiral or spirochetal. [NIH]

Baths: The immersion or washing of the body or any of its parts in water or other medium for cleansing or medical treatment. It includes bathing for personal hygiene as well as for medical purposes with the addition of therapeutic agents, such as alkalines, antiseptics, oil, etc. [NIH]

Benign: Not malignant; not recurrent; favourable for recovery. [EU]

Biliary: Pertaining to the bile, to the bile ducts, or to the gallbladder. [EU]

Bilirubin: A bile pigment that is a degradation product of heme. [NIH]

Bioavailability: The degree to which a drug or other substance becomes available to the target tissue after administration. [EU]

Biochemical: Relating to biochemistry; characterized by, produced by, or involving chemical reactions in living organisms. [EU]

Biopsy: The removal and examination, usually microscopic, of tissue from the living body, performed to establish precise diagnosis. [EU]

Bleomycin: A complex of related glycopeptide antibiotics from Streptomyces verticillus consisting of bleomycin A2 and B2. It inhibits DNA metabolism and is used as an antineoplastic, especially for solid tumors. [NIH]

Bullous: Pertaining to or characterized by bullae. [EU]

Calcinosis: Pathologic deposition of calcium salts in tissues. [NIH]

Camptothecin: An alkaloid isolated from the stem wood of the Chinese tree, Camptotheca acuminata. This compound selectively inhibits the nuclear enzyme DNA topoisomerase. Several semisynthetic analogs of camptothecin have demonstrated antitumor activity. [NIH]

Candidiasis: Infection with a fungus of the genus Candida. It is usually a superficial infection of the moist cutaneous areas of the body, and is generally caused by C. albicans; it most commonly involves the skin (dermatocandidiasis), oral mucous membranes (thrush, def. 1), respiratory tract (bronchocandidiasis), and vagina (vaginitis). Rarely there is a systemic infection or endocarditis. Called also moniliasis, candidosis, oidiomycosis, and formerly blastodendriosis. [EU]

Capillary: Any one of the minute vessels that connect the arterioles and venules, forming a network in nearly all parts of the body. Their walls act as semipermeable membranes for the interchange of various substances, including fluids, between the blood and tissue fluid; called also vas capillare. [EU]

Capsules: Hard or soft soluble containers used for the oral administration of medicine. [NIH]

Captopril: A potent and specific inhibitor of peptidyl-dipeptidase A. It blocks the conversion of angiotensin I to angiotensin II, a vasoconstrictor and important regulator of arterial blood pressure. Captopril acts to suppress the renin-angiotensin system and inhibits pressure responses to exogenous angiotensin. [NIH]

Carbidopa: A peripheral inhibitor of dopa decarboxylase. It is given in parkinsonism along with levodopa to inhibit the conversion of levodopa to dopamine in the periphery, thereby reducing the peripheral adverse effects, increasing the amount of levodopa that reaches the central nervous system, and reducing the dose needed. It has no antiparkinson actions when given alone. [NIH]

Carbohydrate: An aldehyde or ketone derivative of a polyhydric alcohol, particularly of the pentahydric and hexahydric alcohols. They are so named because the hydrogen and oxygen are usually in the proportion to form water, $(CH_2O)n$. The most important carbohydrates are the starches, sugars, celluloses, and gums. They are classified into mono-, di-, tri-, poly- and heterosaccharides. [EU]

Carcinoma: A malignant new growth made up of epithelial cells tending to infiltrate the surrounding tissues and give rise to metastases. [EU]

Cardiac: Pertaining to the heart. [EU]

Cardiomyopathy: A general diagnostic term designating primary myocardial disease, often of obscure or unknown etiology. [EU]

Carotene: The general name for a group of pigments found in green, yellow, and leafy vegetables, and yellow fruits. The pigments are fat-soluble, unsaturated aliphatic hydrocarbons functioning as provitamins and are converted to vitamin A through enzymatic processes in the intestinal wall. [NIH]

Caustic: An escharotic or corrosive agent. Called also cauterant. [EU]

Chemotherapy: The treatment of disease by means of chemicals that have a specific toxic effect upon the disease - producing microorganisms or that selectively destroy cancerous tissue. [EU]

Chloroquine: The prototypical antimalarial agent with a mechanism that is not well understood. It has also been used to treat rheumatoid arthritis, systemic lupus erythematosus, and in the systemic therapy of amebic liver abscesses. [NIH]

Cholesterol: The principal sterol of all higher animals, distributed in body tissues, especially the brain and spinal cord, and in animal fats and oils. [NIH]

Chronic: Persisting over a long period of time. [EU]

Cirrhosis: Liver disease characterized pathologically by loss of the normal microscopic lobular architecture, with fibrosis and nodular regeneration. The term is sometimes used to refer to chronic interstitial inflammation of any organ. [EU]

Clindamycin: An antibacterial agent that is a semisynthetic analog of lincomycin. [NIH]

Coagulation: 1. the process of clot formation. 2. in colloid chemistry, the solidification of a sol into a gelatinous mass; an alteration of a disperse phase or of a dissolved solid which causes the separation of the system into a liquid phase and an insoluble mass called the clot or curd. Coagulation is usually irreversible. 3. in surgery, the disruption of tissue by physical means to form an amorphous residuum, as in electrocoagulation and photocoagulation. [EU]

Colitis: Inflammation of the colon. [EU]

Collagen: The protein substance of the white fibres (collagenous fibres) of skin, tendon, bone, cartilage, and all other connective tissue; composed of molecules of tropocollagen (q.v.), it is converted into gelatin by boiling. collagenous pertaining to collagen; forming or producing collagen. [EU]

Contracture: A condition of fixed high resistance to passive stretch of a muscle, resulting from fibrosis of the tissues supporting the muscles or the joints, or from disorders of the muscle fibres. [EU]

Coronary: Encircling in the manner of a crown; a term applied to vessels; nerves, ligaments, etc. The term usually denotes the arteries that supply the heart muscle and, by extension, a pathologic involvement of them. [EU]

Curcumin: A dye obtained from tumeric, the powdered root of Curcuma longa Linn. It is used in the preparation of curcuma paper and the detection of boron. Curcumin appears to possess a spectrum of pharmacological properties, due primarily to its inhibitory effects on metabolic enzymes. [NIH]

Cutaneous: Pertaining to the skin; dermal; dermic. [EU]

Cyclophosphamide: Precursor of an alkylating nitrogen mustard antineoplastic and immunosuppressive agent that must be activated in the liver to form the active aldophosphamide. It is used in the treatment of lymphomas, leukemias, etc. Its side effect, alopecia, has been made use of in defleecing sheep. Cyclophosphamide may also cause sterility, birth defects, mutations, and cancer. [NIH]

Cytokines: Non-antibody proteins secreted by inflammatory leukocytes and some non-leukocytic cells, that act as intercellular mediators. They differ from classical hormones in that they are produced by a number of tissue or cell types rather than by specialized glands. They generally act locally in a paracrine or autocrine rather than endocrine manner. [NIH]

Cytomegalovirus: A genus of the family herpesviridae, subfamily betaherpesvirinae, infecting the salivary glands, liver, spleen, lungs, eyes, and other organs, in which they produce characteristically enlarged cells with intranuclear inclusions. Infection with Cytomegalovirus is also seen as an opportunistic infection in AIDS. [NIH]

Degenerative: Undergoing degeneration : tending to degenerate; having the character of or involving degeneration; causing or tending to cause degeneration. [EU]

Dehydration: The condition that results from excessive loss of body water. Called also anhydration, deaquation and hypohydration. [EU]

Dentists: Individuals licensed to practice dentistry. [NIH]

Dermatitis: Inflammation of the skin. [EU]

Dermatology: A medical specialty concerned with the skin, its structure, functions, diseases, and treatment. [NIH]

Dermatosis: Any skin disease, especially one not characterized by inflammation. [EU]

Dermis: A layer of vascular connective tissue underneath the epidermis. The surface of the dermis contains sensitive papillae. Embedded in or beneath the dermis are sweat glands, hair follicles, and sebaceous glands. [NIH]

Diffusion: The process of becoming diffused, or widely spread; the spontaneous movement of molecules or other particles in solution, owing to their random thermal motion, to reach a uniform concentration throughout the solvent, a process requiring no addition of energy to the system. [EU]

Digestion: The process of breakdown of food for metabolism and use by the body. [NIH]

Dimethyl Sulfoxide: A highly polar organic liquid, that is used widely as a chemical solvent. Because of its ability to penetrate biological membranes, it is used as a vehicle for topical application of pharmaceuticals. It is also used to protect tissue during cryopreservation. Dimethyl sulfoxide shows a range of pharmacological activity including analgesia and anti-inflammation. [NIH]

Distal: Remote; farther from any point of reference; opposed to proximal. In dentistry, used to designate a position on the dental arch farther from the median line of the jaw. [EU]

Dysphagia: Difficulty in swallowing. [EU]

Dyspnea: Difficult or labored breathing. [NIH]

Dystrophy: Any disorder arising from defective or faulty nutrition, especially the muscular dystrophies. [EU]

Elasticity: Resistance and recovery from distortion of shape. [NIH]

Emollient: Softening or soothing; called also malactic. [EU]

Enalapril: An angiotensin-converting enzyme inhibitor that is used to treat hypertension. [NIH]

Endogenous: Developing or originating within the organisms or arising from causes within the organism. [EU]

Enzyme: A protein molecule that catalyses chemical reactions of other substances without itself being destroyed or altered upon completion of the reactions. Enzymes are classified according to the recommendations of the Nomenclature Committee of the International Union of Biochemistry. Each enzyme is assigned a recommended name and an Enzyme Commission (EC) number. They are divided into six main groups; oxidoreductases, transferases, hydrolases, lyases, isomerases, and ligases. [EU]

Eosinophilia: The formation and accumulation of an abnormally large number of eosinophils in the blood. [EU]

Eosinophils: Granular leukocytes with a nucleus that usually has two lobes connected by a slender thread of chromatin, and cytoplasm containing coarse, round granules that are uniform in size and stainable by eosin. [NIH]

Epidemic: Occurring suddenly in numbers clearly in excess of normal expectancy; said especially of infectious diseases but applied also to any disease, injury, or other health-related event occurring in such outbreaks. [EU]

Epidemiological: Relating to, or involving epidemiology. [EU]

Epidermal: Pertaining to or resembling epidermis. Called also epidermic or epidermoid. [EU]

Epitopes: Sites on an antigen that interact with specific antibodies. [NIH]

Epoprostenol: A prostaglandin that is biosynthesized enzymatically from prostaglandin endoperoxides in human vascular tissue. It is a potent inhibitor of platelet aggregation. The sodium salt has been also used to treat primary pulmonary hypertension. [NIH]

Erythromycin: A bacteriostatic antibiotic substance produced by Streptomyces erythreus. Erythromycin A is considered its major active component. In sensitive organisms, it inhibits protein synthesis by binding to 50S ribosomal subunits. This binding process inhibits peptidyl transferase activity and interferes with translocation of amino acids during translation and assembly of proteins. [NIH]

Esophagitis: Inflammation, acute or chronic, of the esophagus caused by bacteria, chemicals, or trauma. [NIH]

Exogenous: Developed or originating outside the organism, as exogenous disease. [EU]

Extracorporeal: Situated or occurring outside the body. [EU]

Fatigue: The state of weariness following a period of exertion, mental or physical, characterized by a decreased capacity for work and reduced efficiency to respond to stimuli. [NIH]

Febrile: Pertaining to or characterized by fever. [EU]

Fibroblasts: Connective tissue cells which secrete an extracellular matrix rich in collagen and other macromolecules. [NIH]

Fibrosis: The formation of fibrous tissue; fibroid or fibrous degeneration [EU]

Gangrene: Death of tissue, usually in considerable mass and generally associated with loss of vascular (nutritive) supply and followed by bacterial invasion and putrefaction. [EU]

Gastrointestinal: Pertaining to or communicating with the stomach and intestine, as a gastrointestinal fistula. [EU]

Gels: Colloids with a solid continuous phase and liquid as the dispersed phase; gels may be unstable when, due to temperature or other cause, the solid phase liquifies; the resulting colloid is called a sol. [NIH]

Genotype: The genetic constitution of the individual; the characterization of the genes. [NIH]

Gingivitis: Inflammation of the gingivae. Gingivitis associated with bony changes is referred to as periodontitis. Called also oulitis and ulitis. [EU]

Griseofulvin: An antifungal antibiotic. Griseofulvin may be given by mouth in the treatment of tinea infections. [NIH]

Halitosis: An offensive, foul breath odor resulting from a variety of causes such as poor oral hygiene, dental or oral infections, or the ingestion of certain foods. [NIH]

Haplotypes: The genetic constitution of individuals with respect to one member of a pair of allelic genes, or sets of genes that are closely linked and tend to be inherited together such as those of the major histocompatibility complex. [NIH]

Heartburn: Substernal pain or burning sensation, usually associated with regurgitation of gastric juice into the esophagus. [NIH]

Hematocrit: Measurement of the volume of packed red cells in a blood specimen by centrifugation. The procedure is performed using a tube with graduated markings or with automated blood cell counters. It is used as an indicator of erythrocyte status in disease. For example, anemia shows a low hematocrit, polycythemia, high values. [NIH]

Hemorrhage: Bleeding or escape of blood from a vessel. [NIH]

Heredity: 1. the genetic transmission of a particular quality or trait from parent to offspring. 2. the genetic constitution of an individual. [EU]

Herpes: Any inflammatory skin disease caused by a herpesvirus and characterized by the formation of clusters of small vesicles. When used alone, the term may refer to herpes simplex or to herpes zoster. [EU]

Hoarseness: An unnaturally deep or rough quality of voice. [NIH]

Hobbies: Leisure activities engaged in for pleasure. [NIH]

Homologous: Corresponding in structure, position, origin, etc., as (a) the feathers of a bird and the scales of a fish, (b) antigen and its specific antibody, (c) allelic chromosomes. [EU]

Hormones: Chemical substances having a specific regulatory effect on the activity of a certain organ or organs. The term was originally applied to substances secreted by various endocrine glands and transported in the bloodstream to the target organs. It is sometimes extended to include those substances that are not produced by the endocrine glands but that have similar effects. [NIH]

Humoral: Of, relating to, proceeding from, or involving a bodily humour - now often used of endocrine factors as opposed to neural or somatic. [EU]

Hybridization: The genetic process of crossbreeding to produce a hybrid. Hybrid nucleic acids can be formed by nucleic acid hybridization of DNA and RNA molecules. Protein hybridization allows for hybrid proteins to be formed from polypeptide chains. [NIH]

Hydroxyproline: A hydroxylated form of the imino acid proline. A deficiency in ascorbic acid can result in impaired hydroxyproline formation. [NIH]

Hyperbaric: Characterized by greater than normal pressure or weight; applied to gases under greater than atmospheric pressure, as hyperbaric oxygen, or to a solution of greater specific gravity than another taken as a standard of reference. [EU]

Hyperplasia: The abnormal multiplication or increase in the number of normal cells in normal arrangement in a tissue. [EU]

Hypertension: Persistently high arterial blood pressure. Various criteria for its threshold have been suggested, ranging from 140 mm. Hg systolic and 90 mm. Hg diastolic to as high as 200 mm. Hg systolic and 110 mm. Hg diastolic. Hypertension may have no known cause (essential or idiopathic h.) or be associated with other primary diseases (secondary h.). [EU]

Hypopigmentation: A condition caused by a deficiency in melanin formation or a loss of pre-existing melanin or melanocytes. It can be complete or partial and may result from trauma, inflammation, and certain infections. [NIH]

Hypothyroidism: Deficiency of thyroid activity. In adults, it is most common in women and is characterized by decrease in basal metabolic rate, tiredness and lethargy, sensitivity to cold, and menstrual disturbances. If untreated, it progresses to full-blown myxoedema. In infants, severe hypothyroidism leads to cretinism. In juveniles, the manifestations are intermediate, with less severe mental and developmental retardation and only mild symptoms of the adult form. When due to pituitary deficiency of thyrotropin secretion it is called secondary hypothyroidism. [EU]

Idiopathic: Of the nature of an idiopathy; self-originated; of unknown causation. [EU]

Iloprost: An eicosanoid, derived from the cyclooxygenase pathway of arachidonic acid metabolism. It is a stable and synthetic analog of epoprostenol, but with a longer half-life than the parent compound. Its actions are similar to prostacyclin. Iloprost produces vasodilation and inhibits platelet aggregation. [NIH]

Immunochemistry: Field of chemistry that pertains to immunological phenomena and the study of chemical reactions related to antigen stimulation of tissues. It includes physicochemical interactions between antigens and antibodies. [NIH]

Impotence: The inability to perform sexual intercourse. [NIH]

Induction: The act or process of inducing or causing to occur, especially the production of a specific morphogenetic effect in the developing embryo through the influence of evocators or organizers, or the production of anaesthesia or unconsciousness by use of appropriate agents. [EU]

Induration: 1. the quality of being hard; the process of hardening. 2. an abnormally hard spot or place. [EU]

Infiltration: The diffusion or accumulation in a tissue or cells of substances not normal to it or in amounts of the normal. Also, the material so accumulated. [EU]

Inflammation: A pathological process characterized by injury or destruction of tissues caused by a variety of cytologic and chemical reactions. It is usually manifested by typical signs of pain, heat, redness, swelling, and loss of function. [NIH]

Infusion: The therapeutic introduction of a fluid other than blood, as saline solution, solution, into a vein. [EU]

Ingestion: The act of taking food, medicines, etc., into the body, by mouth. [EU]

Interferons: Proteins secreted by vertebrate cells in response to a wide variety of inducers. They confer resistance against many different viruses, inhibit proliferation of normal and malignant cells, impede multiplication of intracellular parasites, enhance macrophage and granulocyte phagocytosis, augment natural killer cell activity, and show several other immunomodulatory functions. [NIH]

Interleukins: Soluble factors which stimulate growth-related activities of leukocytes as well as other cell types. They enhance cell proliferation and differentiation, DNA synthesis, secretion of other biologically active molecules and responses to immune and inflammatory stimuli. [NIH]

Interstitial: Pertaining to or situated between parts or in the interspaces of a tissue. [EU]

Intestines: The section of the alimentary canal from the stomach to the anus. It includes the large intestine and small intestine. [NIH]

Invasive: 1. having the quality of invasiveness. 2. involving puncture or incision of the skin or insertion of an instrument or foreign material into the body; said of diagnostic techniques. [EU]

Iodine: A nonmetallic element of the halogen group that is represented by the atomic symbol I, atomic number 53, and atomic weight of 126.90. It is a nutritionally essential element, especially important in thyroid hormone synthesis. In solution, it has anti-infective properties and is used topically. [NIH]

Ischemia: Deficiency of blood in a part, due to functional constriction or actual obstruction of a blood vessel. [EU]

Keratoconjunctivitis: Inflammation of the cornea and conjunctiva. [EU]

Keratosis: Any horny growth such as a wart or callus. [NIH]

Kinetic: Pertaining to or producing motion. [EU]

Kinetochores: Large multiprotein complexes that bind the centromeres of the chromosomes to the microtubules of the mitotic spindle during metaphase in the cell cycle. [NIH]

Lacrimal: Pertaining to the tears. [EU]

Larynx: An irregularly shaped, musculocartilaginous tubular structure, lined with mucous membrane, located at the top of the trachea and below the root of the tongue and the hyoid bone. It is the essential sphincter guarding the entrance into the trachea and functioning secondarily as the organ of voice. [NIH]

Lesion: Any pathological or traumatic discontinuity of tissue or loss of function of a part. [EU]

Leukapheresis: The preparation of leukocyte concentrates with the return of red cells and leukocyte-poor plasma to the donor. [NIH]

Levodopa: The naturally occurring form of dopa and the immediate precursor of dopamine. Unlike dopamine itself, it can be taken orally and crosses the blood-brain barrier. It is rapidly taken up by dopaminergic neurons and converted to dopamine. It is used for the treatment of parkinsonism and is usually given with agents that inhibit its conversion to dopamine outside of the central nervous system. [NIH]

Ligament: A band of fibrous tissue that connects bones or cartilages, serving to support and strengthen joints. [EU]

Ligation: Application of a ligature to tie a vessel or strangulate a part. [NIH]

Lip: Either of the two fleshy, full-blooded margins of the mouth. [NIH]

Lubrication: The application of a substance to diminish friction between two surfaces. It may refer to oils, greases, and similar substances for the lubrication of medical equipment but it can be used for the application of substances to tissue to reduce friction, such as lotions for skin and vaginal lubricants. [NIH]

Lupus: A form of cutaneous tuberculosis. It is seen predominantly in women and typically involves the nasal, buccal, and conjunctival mucosa. [NIH]

Lymphoma: Any neoplastic disorder of the lymphoid tissue, the term lymphoma often is used alone to denote malignant lymphoma. [EU]

Malabsorption: Impaired intestinal absorption of nutrients. [EU]

Malformation: A morphologic defect resulting from an intrinsically abnormal developmental process. [EU]

Malignant: Tending to become progressively worse and to result in death. Having the properties of anaplasia, invasion, and metastasis; said of tumours. [EU]

Mediator: An object or substance by which something is mediated, such as (1) a structure of the nervous system that transmits impulses eliciting a specific response; (2) a chemical substance (transmitter substance) that induces activity in an excitable tissue, such as nerve or muscle; or (3) a substance released from cells as the result of the interaction of antigen with antibody or by the action of antigen with a sensitized lymphocyte. [EU]

Membrane: A thin layer of tissue which covers a surface, lines a cavity or divides a space or organ. [EU]

Methotrexate: An antineoplastic antimetabolite with immunosuppressant properties. It is an inhibitor of dihydrofolate reductase and prevents the formation of tetrahydrofolate, necessary for synthesis of thymidylate, an essential component of DNA. [NIH]

Microgram: A unit of mass (weight) of the metric system, being one-millionth of a gram (10-6 gm.) or one one-thousandth of a milligram (10-3 mg.). [EU]

Microscopy: The application of microscope magnification to the study of materials that cannot be properly seen by the unaided eye. [NIH]

Molecular: Of, pertaining to, or composed of molecules : a very small mass of matter. [EU]

Monocytes: Large, phagocytic mononuclear leukocytes produced in the vertebrate bone marrow and released into the blood; contain a large, oval or somewhat indented nucleus surrounded by voluminous cytoplasm and numerous organelles. [NIH]

Mutagenesis: Process of generating genetic mutations. It may occur spontaneously or be induced by mutagens. [NIH]

Myalgia: Pain in a muscle or muscles. [EU]

Mycosis: Any disease caused by a fungus. [EU]

Myeloma: A tumour composed of cells of the type normally found in the bone marrow. [EU]

Myocarditis: Inflammation of the myocardium; inflammation of the muscular walls of the heart. [EU]

Myositis: Inflammation of a voluntary muscle. [EU]

Nausea: An unpleasant sensation, vaguely referred to the epigastrium and abdomen, and often culminating in vomiting. [EU]

Necrosis: The sum of the morphological changes indicative of cell death and caused by the progressive degradative action of enzymes; it may affect groups of cells or part of a structure or an organ. [EU]

Neonatal: Pertaining to the first four weeks after birth. [EU]

Neural: 1. pertaining to a nerve or to the nerves. 2. situated in the region of the spinal axis, as the neutral arch. [EU]

Neurologic: Pertaining to neurology or to the nervous system. [EU]

Niacin: Water-soluble vitamin of the B complex occurring in various animal and plant tissues. Required by the body for the formation of coenzymes NAD and NADP. Has pellagra-curative, vasodilating, and antilipemic properties. [NIH]

Nifedipine: A potent vasodilator agent with calcium antagonistic action. It is a useful anti-anginal agent that also lowers blood pressure. The use of nifedipine as a tocolytic is being investigated. [NIH]

Nitrogen: An element with the atomic symbol N, atomic number 7, and atomic weight 14. Nitrogen exists as a diatomic gas and makes up about 78% of the earth's atmosphere by volume. It is a constituent of proteins and nucleic acids and found in all living cells. [NIH]

Ophthalmic: Pertaining to the eye. [EU]

Oral: Pertaining to the mouth, taken through or applied in the mouth, as an oral medication or an oral thermometer. [EU]

Osteoporosis: Reduction in the amount of bone mass, leading to fractures after minimal trauma. [EU]

Overdose: 1. to administer an excessive dose. 2. an excessive dose. [EU]

Oxidation: The act of oxidizing or state of being oxidized. Chemically it consists in the increase of positive charges on an atom or the loss of negative charges. Most biological oxidations are accomplished by the removal of a pair of hydrogen atoms (dehydrogenation) from a molecule. Such oxidations must be accompanied by reduction of an acceptor molecule. Univalent o. indicates loss of one electron; divalent o., the loss of two electrons. [EU]

Parasitic: Pertaining to, of the nature of, or caused by a parasite. [EU]

Parenteral: Not through the alimentary canal but rather by injection through some other route, as subcutaneous, intramuscular, intraorbital, intracapsular, intraspinal, intrasternal, intravenous, etc. [EU]

Penicillamine: 3-Mercapto-D-valine. The most characteristic degradation product of the penicillin antibiotics. It is used as an antirheumatic and as a chelating agent in Wilson's disease. [NIH]

Perforation: 1. the act of boring or piercing through a part. 2. a hole made through a part or substance. [EU]

Perioral: Situated or occurring around the mouth. [EU]

Perivascular: Situated around a vessel. [EU]

Pharmacologic: Pertaining to pharmacology or to the properties and reactions of drugs. [EU]

Phenytoin: An anticonvulsant that is used in a wide variety of seizures. It is also an anti-arrhythmic and a muscle relaxant. The mechanism of therapeutic action is not clear, although several cellular actions have been described including effects on ion channels, active transport, and general membrane stabilization. The mechanism of its muscle relaxant effect appears to involve a reduction in the sensitivity of muscle spindles to stretch. Phenytoin has been proposed for several other therapeutic uses, but its use has been limited by its many adverse effects and interactions with other drugs. [NIH]

Phosphorylation: The introduction of a phosphoryl group into a compound through the formation of an ester bond between the compound and a phosphorus moiety. [NIH]

Photochemotherapy: Therapy using oral or topical photosensitizing agents with subsequent exposure to light. [NIH]

Phototherapy: Treatment of disease by exposure to light, especially by variously concentrated light rays or specific wavelengths. [NIH]

Pigmentation: 1. the deposition of colouring matter; the coloration or discoloration of a part by pigment. 2. coloration, especially abnormally increased coloration, by melanin. [EU]

Pilocarpine: A slowly hydrolyzed muscarinic agonist with no nicotinic effects. Pilocarpine is used as a miotic and in the treatment of glaucoma. [NIH]

Placenta: A highly vascular fetal organ through which the fetus absorbs oxygen and other nutrients and excretes carbon dioxide and other wastes. It begins to form about the eighth day of gestation when the blastocyst adheres to the decidua. [NIH]

Pneumonia: Inflammation of the lungs with consolidation. [EU]

Polypeptide: A peptide which on hydrolysis yields more than two amino acids; called tripeptides, tetrapeptides, etc. according to the number of amino acids contained. [EU]

Porphyria: A pathological state in man and some lower animals that is often due to genetic factors, is characterized by abnormalities of porphyrin metabolism, and results in the excretion of large quantities of porphyrins in the urine and in extreme sensitivity to light. [EU]

Predisposition: A latent susceptibility to disease which may be activated under certain conditions, as by stress. [EU]

Prednisone: A synthetic anti-inflammatory glucocorticoid derived from cortisone. It is biologically inert and converted to prednisolone in the liver. [NIH]

Prevalence: The total number of cases of a given disease in a specified population at a designated time. It is differentiated from incidence, which refers to the number of new cases in the population at a given time. [NIH]

Procollagen: A biosynthetic precursor of collagen containing additional amino acid sequences at the amino-terminal ends of the three polypeptide chains. Protocollagen, a precursor of procollagen consists of procollagen peptide chains in which proline and lysine have not yet been hydroxylated. [NIH]

Progeria: An abnormal congenital condition characterized by premature aging in children, where all the changes of cell senescence occur. It is manifested by premature greying, hair loss, hearing loss, cataracts, arthritis,osteoporosis, diabetes mellitus, atrophy of subcutaneous fat, skeletal hypoplasia, and accelerated atherosclerosis. Many affected individuals develop malignant tumors, especially sarcomas. [NIH]

Progressive: Advancing; going forward; going from bad to worse; increasing in scope or severity. [EU]

Proportional: Being in proportion : corresponding in size, degree, or intensity, having the same or a constant ratio; of, relating to, or used in determining proportions. [EU]

Prostaglandins: A group of compounds derived from unsaturated 20-carbon fatty acids, primarily arachidonic acid, via the cyclooxygenase pathway. They are extremely potent mediators of a diverse group of physiological processes. [NIH]

Protease: Proteinase (= any enzyme that catalyses the splitting of interior peptide bonds in a protein). [EU]

Proteins: Polymers of amino acids linked by peptide bonds. The specific sequence of amino acids determines the shape and function of the protein. [NIH]

Proximal: Nearest; closer to any point of reference; opposed to distal. [EU]

Pruritus: 1. itching; an unpleasant cutaneous sensation that provokes the desire to rub or scratch the skin to obtain relief. 2. any of various conditions marked by itching, the specific site or type being indicated by a modifying term. [EU]

Psoriasis: A common genetically determined, chronic, inflammatory skin disease characterized by rounded erythematous, dry, scaling patches. The lesions have a predilection for nails, scalp, genitalia, extensor surfaces, and the lumbosacral region. Accelerated epidermopoiesis is considered to be the fundamental pathologic feature in psoriasis. [NIH]

Pulmonary: Pertaining to the lungs. [EU]

Purpura: Purplish or brownish red discoloration, easily visible through the epidermis, caused by hemorrhage into the tissues. [NIH]

Radiology: A specialty concerned with the use of x-ray and other forms of radiant energy in the diagnosis and treatment of disease. [NIH]

Reagent: A substance employed to produce a chemical reaction so as to detect, measure, produce, etc., other substances. [EU]

Receptor: 1. a molecular structure within a cell or on the surface characterized by (1) selective binding of a specific substance and (2) a specific physiologic effect that accompanies the binding, e.g., cell-surface receptors for peptide hormones, neurotransmitters, antigens, complement fragments, and immunoglobulins and cytoplasmic receptors for steroid hormones. 2. a sensory nerve terminal that responds to stimuli of various kinds. [EU]

Recombinant: 1. a cell or an individual with a new combination of genes not found together in either parent; usually applied to linked genes. [EU]

Reconstitution: 1. a type of regeneration in which a new organ forms by the rearrangement of tissues rather than from new formation at an injured surface. 2. the restoration to original form of a substance previously altered for preservation and storage, as the restoration to a liquid state of blood serum or plasma that has been dried and stored. [EU]

Recurrence: The return of a sign, symptom, or disease after a remission. [NIH]

Reflective: Capable of throwing back light, images, sound waves: reflecting. [EU]

Reflux: A backward or return flow. [EU]

Refractory: Not readily yielding to treatment. [EU]

Reserpine: An alkaloid found in the roots of Rauwolfia serpentina and R. vomitoria. Reserpine inhibits the uptake of norepinephrine into storage vesicles resulting in depletion of catecholamines and serotonin from central and peripheral axon terminals. It has been used as an antihypertensive and an antipsychotic as well as a research tool, but its adverse effects limit its clinical use. [NIH]

Resorption: The loss of substance through physiologic or pathologic means, such as loss of dentin and cementum of a tooth, or of the alveolar process of the mandible or maxilla. [EU]

Retinoids: Derivatives of vitamin A. Used clinically in the treatment of severe cystic acne, psoriasis, and other disorders of keratinization. Their possible use in the prophylaxis and treatment of cancer is being actively explored. [NIH]

Rheumatoid: Resembling rheumatism. [EU]

Rheumatology: A subspecialty of internal medicine concerned with the study of inflammatory or degenerative processes and metabolic derangement of connective tissue structures which pertain to a variety of musculoskeletal disorders, such as arthritis. [NIH]

Riboflavin: Nutritional factor found in milk, eggs, malted barley, liver, kidney, heart, and leafy vegetables. The richest natural source is yeast. It occurs in the free form only in the retina of the eye, in whey, and in urine; its principal forms in tissues and cells are as FMN and FAD. [NIH]

Sarcoidosis: An idiopathic systemic inflammatory granulomatous disorder comprised of epithelioid and multinucleated giant cells with little necrosis. It usually invades the lungs with fibrosis and may also involve lymph nodes, skin, liver, spleen, eyes, phalangeal bones, and parotid glands. [NIH]

Sclerosis: A induration, or hardening; especially hardening of a part from inflammation and in diseases of the interstitial substance. The term is used chiefly for such a hardening of the nervous system due to hyperplasia of the connective tissue or to designate hardening of the blood vessels. [EU]

Secretion: 1. the process of elaborating a specific product as a result of the activity of a gland; this activity may range from separating a specific substance of the blood to the elaboration of a new chemical substance. 2. any substance produced by secretion. [EU]

Selenium: An element with the atomic symbol Se, atomic number 34, and atomic weight 78.96. It is an essential micronutrient for mammals and other animals but is toxic in large amounts. Selenium protects intracellular structures against oxidative damage. It is an essential component of glutathione peroxidase. [NIH]

Serum: The clear portion of any body fluid; the clear fluid moistening serous membranes. 2. blood serum; the clear liquid that separates from blood on clotting. 3. immune serum; blood serum from an immunized animal used for passive immunization; an antiserum; antitoxin, or antivenin. [EU]

Sialorrhea: Increased salivary flow. [NIH]

Silver Sulfadiazine: Antibacterial used topically in burn therapy. [NIH]

Soaps: Sodium or potassium salts of long chain fatty acids. These detergent substances are obtained by boiling natural oils or fats with caustic alkali. Sodium soaps are harder and are used as topical anti-infectives and vehicles in pills and liniments; potassium soaps are soft, used as vehicles for ointments and also as topical antimicrobials. [NIH]

Solvent: 1. dissolving; effecting a solution. 2. a liquid that dissolves or that is capable of dissolving; the component of a solution that is present in greater amount. [EU]

Spectrum: A charted band of wavelengths of electromagnetic vibrations obtained by refraction and diffraction. By extension, a measurable range of activity, such as the range of bacteria affected by an antibiotic (antibacterial s.) or the complete range of manifestations of a disease. [EU]

Spondylitis: Inflammation of the vertebrae. [EU]

Stasis: A word termination indicating the maintenance of (or maintaining) a constant level; preventing increase or multiplication. [EU]

Stomach: An organ of digestion situated in the left upper quadrant of the abdomen between the termination of the esophagus and the beginning of the duodenum. [NIH]

Stomatitis: Inflammation of the oral mucosa, due to local or systemic factors which may involve the buccal and labial mucosa, palate, tongue, floor of the mouth, and the gingivae. [EU]

Sunburn: An injury to the skin causing erythema, tenderness, and sometimes blistering and resulting from excessive exposure to the sun. The reaction is produced by the ultraviolet radiation in sunlight. [NIH]

Sweat: The fluid excreted by the sweat glands. It consists of water containing sodium chloride, phosphate, urea, ammonia, and other waste products. [NIH]

Symptomatic: 1. pertaining to or of the nature of a symptom. 2. indicative (of a particular disease or disorder). 3. exhibiting the symptoms of a particular disease but having a different cause. 4. directed at the allying of symptoms, as symptomatic treatment. [EU]

Systemic: Pertaining to or affecting the body as a whole. [EU]

Teratogenic: Tending to produce anomalies of formation, or teratism (= anomaly of formation or development : condition of a monster). [EU]

Thalidomide: A pharmaceutical agent originally introduced as a non-barbiturate hypnotic, but withdrawn from the market because of its known tetratogenic effects. It has been reintroduced and used for a number of immunological and inflammatory disorders. Thalidomide displays immunosuppresive and anti-angiogenic activity. It inhibits release of tumor necrosis factor alpha from monocytes, and modulates other cytokine action. [NIH]

Thermal: Pertaining to or characterized by heat. [EU]

Thermography: Measurement of the regional temperature of the body or an organ by infrared sensing devices, based on self-emanating infrared radiation. [NIH]

Thyrotropin: A peptide hormone secreted by the anterior pituitary. It promotes the growth of the thyroid gland and stimulates the synthesis of thyroid hormones and the release of thyroxine by the thyroid gland. [NIH]

Thyroxine: An amino acid of the thyroid gland which exerts a stimulating effect on thyroid metabolism. [NIH]

Tolerance: 1. the ability to endure unusually large doses of a drug or toxin. 2. acquired drug tolerance; a decreasing response to repeated constant doses of a drug or the need for increasing doses to maintain a constant response. [EU]

Tomography: The recording of internal body images at a predetermined plane by means of the tomograph; called also body section roentgenography. [EU]

Topical: Pertaining to a particular surface area, as a topical anti-infective applied to a certain area of the skin and affecting only the area to which it is applied. [EU]

Toxic: Pertaining to, due to, or of the nature of a poison or toxin;

manifesting the symptoms of severe infection. [EU]

Toxicity: The quality of being poisonous, especially the degree of virulence of a toxic microbe or of a poison. [EU]

Transcutaneous: Transdermal. [EU]

Transfusion: The introduction of whole blood or blood component directly into the blood stream. [EU]

Transplantation: The grafting of tissues taken from the patient's own body or from another. [EU]

Trichloroethylene: A highly volatile inhalation anesthetic used mainly in short surgical procedures where light anesthesia with good analgesia is required. It is also used as an industrial solvent. Prolonged exposure to high concentrations of the vapor can lead to cardiotoxicity and neurological impairment. [NIH]

Ulcer: A local defect, or excavation, of the surface of an organ or tissue; which is produced by the sloughing of inflammatory necrotic tissue. [EU]

Ulceration: 1. the formation or development of an ulcer. 2. an ulcer. [EU]

Urinalysis: Examination of urine by chemical, physical, or microscopic means. Routine urinalysis usually includes performing chemical screening tests, determining specific gravity, observing any unusual color or odor, screening for bacteriuria, and examining the sediment microscopically. [NIH]

Urticaria: Pathology: a transient condition of the skin, usually caused by an allergic reaction, characterized by pale or reddened irregular, elevated patches and severe itching; hives. [EU]

Vaccine: A suspension of attenuated or killed microorganisms (bacteria, viruses, or rickettsiae), administered for the prevention, amelioration or treatment of infectious diseases. [EU]

Vaginal: 1. of the nature of a sheath; ensheathing. 2. pertaining to the vagina. 3. pertaining to the tunica vaginalis testis. [EU]

Vascular: Pertaining to blood vessels or indicative of a copious blood supply. [EU]

Vasculitis: Inflammation of a vessel, angiitis. [EU]

Vasoactive: Exerting an effect upon the calibre of blood vessels. [EU]

Ventricular: Pertaining to a ventricle. [EU]

Vesicular: 1. composed of or relating to small, saclike bodies. 2. pertaining to or made up of vesicles on the skin. [EU]

Viral: Pertaining to, caused by, or of the nature of virus. [EU]

Viruses: Minute infectious agents whose genomes are composed of DNA or RNA, but not both. They are characterized by a lack of independent metabolism and the inability to replicate outside living host cells. [NIH]

Vitiligo: A disorder consisting of areas of macular depigmentation, commonly on extensor aspects of extremities, on the face or neck, and in skin folds. Age of onset is often in young adulthood and the condition tends to progress gradually with lesions enlarging and extending until a quiescent state is reached. [NIH]

General Dictionaries and Glossaries

While the above glossary is essentially complete, the dictionaries listed here cover virtually all aspects of medicine, from basic words and phrases to more advanced terms (sorted alphabetically by title; hyperlinks provide rankings, information and reviews at Amazon.com):

- **Dictionary of Medical Acronymns & Abbreviations** by Stanley Jablonski (Editor), Paperback, 4th edition (2001), Lippincott Williams & Wilkins Publishers, ISBN: 1560534605,
  http://www.amazon.com/exec/obidos/ASIN/1560534605/icongroupinterna

- **Dictionary of Medical Terms : For the Nonmedical Person (Dictionary of Medical Terms for the Nonmedical Person, Ed 4)** by Mikel A. Rothenberg, M.D, et al, Paperback - 544 pages, 4th edition (2000), Barrons Educational Series, ISBN: 0764112015,
  http://www.amazon.com/exec/obidos/ASIN/0764112015/icongroupinterna

- **A Dictionary of the History of Medicine** by A. Sebastian, CD-Rom edition (2001), CRC Press-Parthenon Publishers, ISBN: 185070368X,
  http://www.amazon.com/exec/obidos/ASIN/185070368X/icongroupinterna

- **Dorland's Illustrated Medical Dictionary (Standard Version)** by Dorland, et al, Hardcover - 2088 pages, 29th edition (2000), W B Saunders Co, ISBN: 0721662544,
  http://www.amazon.com/exec/obidos/ASIN/0721662544/icongroupinterna

- **Dorland's Electronic Medical Dictionary** by Dorland, et al, Software, 29th Book & CD-Rom edition (2000), Harcourt Health Sciences, ISBN: 0721694934,
  http://www.amazon.com/exec/obidos/ASIN/0721694934/icongroupinterna

- **Dorland's Pocket Medical Dictionary (Dorland's Pocket Medical Dictionary, 26th Ed)** Hardcover - 912 pages, 26th edition (2001), W B Saunders Co, ISBN: 0721682812,
  http://www.amazon.com/exec/obidos/ASIN/0721682812/icongroupinterna /103-4193558-7304618

- **Melloni's Illustrated Medical Dictionary (Melloni's Illustrated Medical Dictionary, 4th Ed)** by Melloni, Hardcover, 4th edition (2001), CRC Press-Parthenon Publishers, ISBN: 85070094X,
http://www.amazon.com/exec/obidos/ASIN/85070094X/icongroupinterna

- **Stedman's Electronic Medical Dictionary Version 5.0 (CD-ROM for Windows and Macintosh, Individual)** by Stedmans, CD-ROM edition (2000), Lippincott Williams & Wilkins Publishers, ISBN: 0781726328,
http://www.amazon.com/exec/obidos/ASIN/0781726328/icongroupinterna

- **Stedman's Medical Dictionary** by Thomas Lathrop Stedman, Hardcover - 2098 pages, 27th edition (2000), Lippincott, Williams & Wilkins, ISBN: 068340007X,
http://www.amazon.com/exec/obidos/ASIN/068340007X/icongroupinterna

- **Tabers Cyclopedic Medical Dictionary (Thumb Index)** by Donald Venes (Editor), et al, Hardcover - 2439 pages, 19th edition (2001), F A Davis Co, ISBN: 0803606540,
http://www.amazon.com/exec/obidos/ASIN/0803606540/icongroupinterna

INDEX

Printed in the United States
117168LV00003B/17/A